Textbook of
in vitro Practical Pharmacology

Ian Kitchen
BSc, PhD
Lecturer in Pharmacology
Department of Biochemistry
University of Surrey

BLACKWELL SCIENTIFIC PUBLICATIONS
OXFORD LONDON EDINBURGH
BOSTON MELBOURNE

© 1984 by Blackwell Scientific
  Publications
Editorial offices:
Osney Mead, Oxford, OX2 0EL
8 John Street, London, WC1N 2ES
9 Forrest Road, Edinburgh, EH1 2QH
52 Beacon Street, Boston,
  Massachusetts 02108, USA
99 Barry Street, Carlton, Victoria 3053,
  Australia

First published 1984

Set, printed and bound in Great Britain
by Butler & Tanner Ltd
Frome and London

DISTRIBUTORS

USA
  Blackwell Mosby Book Distributors
  11830 Westline Industrial Drive,
  St Louis, Missouri 63141

Canada
  Blackwell Mosby Book Distributors
  120 Melford Drive, Scarborough,
  Ontario, M1B 2X4

Australia
  Blackwell Scientific Book Distributors
  31 Advantage Road, Highett,
  Victoria 3190

British Library
Cataloguing in Publication Data

Kitchen, Ian
  Textbook of in vitro practical
  pharmacology.
  1. Pharmacology—Laboratory
  manuals
  I. Title
  615'.1'028   RM303

ISBN 0-632-01216-1

Contents

Preface

The most recent textbook covering experiments on isolated preparations was published over thirteen years ago. Since that time a great deal has happened in the field of *in vitro* practical pharmacology which has led me to write this new textbook. The advent of several new isolated tissue preparations in pharmacological research has filtered through to undergraduate teaching of pharmacology. The book therefore includes important additions to the traditional isolated tissues, such as the vas deferens, the anococcygeus and the taenia caeci muscles. In addition, the last decade has seen enormous growth in the use of electronic pharmacological recorders and transducers in the undergraduate teaching laboratory. Accordingly, the book contains an introductory section which includes details of operation of this relatively new teaching equipment. I hope this will be of value not only to the undergraduate pharmacologist but also to postgraduates who embark on research with isolated tissues and have only limited experience in this field. The postgraduate using isolated tissues for the first time may also find the fault-finding section helpful!

Each section of experiments is preceded by tabulated data of experimental parameters and dosages of drugs used. I hope these will be particularly useful for technicians involved in the setting up of practical classes and also as a quick reference source for lecturers involved in practical teaching.

Whilst the use of *in vivo* experiments for teaching pharmacology has been declining in recent years on academic, financial and ethical grounds, *in vitro* practical pharmacology is being retained and often expanded, with the possible exception of the pharmacology taught to medical students. Many medical colleges are now moving towards the use of videotaped practicals. Whilst I feel this is a useful medium, and one which I use myself, there is no substitute for some of the experiments included in this book. For example, the chance to see a fibrillating heart, first hand, is invaluable to the student of medicine. There is of course also the danger of drug response becoming stereotyped. Those involved in the teaching of *in vitro* and *in vivo* pharmacology know only too well that there is no such thing as a 'typical' drug response. This book is therefore aimed at all students who participate in practical pharmacology including medics, pharmacists and pharmacologists.

Three experiments in this book (Expt. 1, 4.7 and 6.6) have preliminary procedures which involve injections of drugs. These procedures require a Home Office Licence in the United Kingdom and must only be carried out by a Home Office Licence holder, covered by the appropriate certificates.

I have compiled this book from my involvement in the teaching of practical pharmacology at Chelsea College, North East London Polytechnic, two London medical schools (St Mary's and The London) and currently at the University of Surrey. I am grateful to the staff of these institutions for their help in the writing of the book and for the use of some of their teaching schedules. Each series of experiments has, where appropriate, photographic illustrations to aid dissection of tissues and also traces of typical responses of each preparation. I would like to thank John Darbey (AVA Unit, Surrey) for his expert photographic work, Paul Green for his assistance in setting up preparations and Dr Margaret Orchard and Julia McDowell for providing me with some of the traces.

The photographs of transducers, electrodes, stimulators and recording apparatus were provided by Harvard Apparatus, Grass Instruments and Ormed. I am grateful for their interest and help.

I would also like to express my thanks to Dr David Burleigh at The London Hospital Medical College for the criticisms and corrections of the manuscript and to Mrs Valerie Saunders for typing countless drafts. In connection with this I perhaps should add my thanks to the word processor. This book would not have been written without it.

Finally, I hope that the errors and omissions are few. I would welcome any comments or criticisms.

1983   I.K.

Introduction

1 General methodology

The methods employed in the use of isolated tissue preparations in practical pharmacology have changed somewhat in recent years, due to the introduction of more sophisticated equipment. It is becoming less common to see the traditional set-up of tissue baths, immersed in water contained within a perspex outer bath and heated by an open water circulator. In its place, both warming coils for the physiological salt solutions and the tissue baths have outer chambers and are heated by water circulators in a closed circuit. It is also clear that the days of the pivoted lever writing on a Kymograph drum, for recording movements of isolated tissues, are numbered. Details of the levers used in pharmacological experiments may be found elsewhere (Edinburgh University Pharmacology Staff, 1968). Many University and Polytechnic departments are now employing isotonic and isometric transducers coupled to an appropriate amplifier and recorder and the use of such equipment will undoubtedly increase. A detailed description of these pharmacological recorders and their operation is provided in section 3.

The viability of isolated tissues varies enormously. Some are extremely robust, are tolerant to over zealous handling and can withstand long periods without oxygen. Others, especially nervous tissue and cardiac muscle, require extremely careful manipulation and will not remain viable for long in the absence of oxygen. In general, it is best to treat all isolated preparations with respect, avoiding stretching of the tissue. Careful attachment to the tissue holder and correct loading of the transducer to give the recommended resting tension are also important. The use of dissecting instruments, especially forceps, should be kept to a minimum, and fingers should be used where possible. It is also worthy of note that ink used in recording apparatus is particularly toxic to many tissues.

I

2 Experimental parameters

Each section of experiments in this book is preceded by a summary of experimental parameters and drugs used in the experiments. The following sections give more detailed elucidation of each of these parameters.

2.1 Organ baths

A guide to the internal volume of organ (or tissue) baths required for each *in vitro* preparation is given throughout the book. For the majority of tissues this is not critical. There are, however, a few exceptions. Where transmural or field stimulation is to be used the dimensions of the organ bath will have an effect on the current passed and it is important not to exceed the recommended volume. The converse is true in experiments where additional apparatus is needed alongside the tissue (e.g. Finkleman preparation, Expt. 2.4). In this case the recommended volumes should not be reduced or the tissue will not be free to move within the bath.

The style of organ bath varies slightly from laboratory to laboratory, but basically consists of an internal chamber with an inflow and outflow for physiological salt solutions and a scinter glass at its base to allow aeration. This is jacketed by an outer warming jacket. The salt solution is fed through a coil which is also contained in a warming jacket. This coil is sometimes integrated within the outer chamber of the organ bath (Fig. 1).

The tissue is secured within the bath either on an internal hook located at the base or on a removable tissue holder. Where there is an internal hook the tissue must be attached by means of a loop tied at one end. The tissue holder has the advantage that the preparation can be securely tied to the hook on the holder's tip. Some purists would claim that only loops are acceptable as this allows the tissue total freedom of movement. Experience has indicated to the author that there is no difference whether loops or ties are used. The author favours the latter since loops have a habit of working free just at a crucial moment.

The need for washing of preparations varies and special instructions related to this are given in individual experiments. Some preparations are more suitably washed by overflow than drainage. This especially includes certain nerve muscle preparations and those muscles which exhibit spontaneous activity when exposed to air. In general a thorough wash should be given before equilibration, and regular washout periods should be maintained throughout the experimental period. Apparatus should always be washed with distilled water after use to prevent the growth of micro-organisms, and periodically cleaned with hydrochloric or chromic acid.

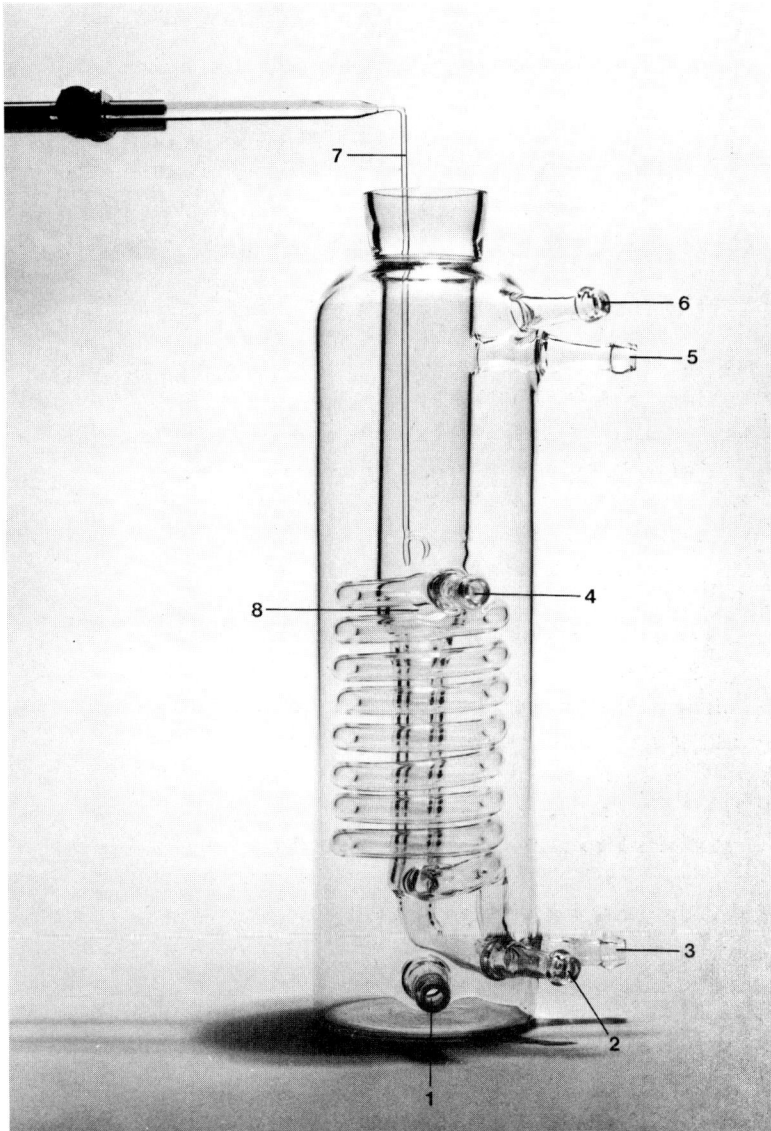

Fig. 1. Typical integrated coil organ bath.

1 Water circulator inflow for outer bath	5 Ringer outflow for washing by over-flow
2 Aeration inflow for inner bath	
3 Ringer outflow	6 Water circulator outflow for outer bath
4 Ringer inflow	7 Tissue holder
	8 Scinter for aeration of inner bath

2.2 Physiological salt solutions

These are often referred to as 'Ringers' after their discoverer Sydney Ringer, in the latter part of the nineteenth century. Table 1 gives the formulae for the solutions described in this book. All solutions are prepared in distilled water and the salts freshly weighed out. Some Pharmacology Departments use stock solutions of some salts, but prolonged storage is not recommended. Although physiological salt solutions may be kept for about 24 hours if stored in the fridge, because of the problems of microbial growth, fresh solutions are always preferable. Calcium chloride should be added last, and as a solution, to prevent precipitation of the bicarbonate. Cloudy solutions will result in non-viable tissues. The two most commonly used solutions are Tyrode and Krebs. As a general rule Tyrode may be used for experiments with non-innervated muscle whilst Krebs is used for nerve muscle preparations. All physiological salt solutions require aeration, either with an air pump, with carbogen ($95\% \ O_2/5\% \ CO_2$) or with oxygen depending on the salt solution used. The buffering capacity of Krebs, for example, is completed by the $5\% \ CO_2$ used in aeration bringing the solution pH to 7.4.

The majority of experiments in this book use mammalian tissues and the salt solution is warmed to the physiological temperature of 37°C. This may be reduced in some experiments for one of two reasons, either to reduce spontaneous movement of the preparation and therefore allow easier estimation of drug induced movement, or to reduce the tissue requirement for oxygen and thereby prolong the viability of the preparation (e.g. cardiac and nerve muscle preparations). The experiments involving amphibian tissue are carried out at room temperature.

2.3 Recording transducers

Many of the pharmacological experiments described require measurements of changes in length or tension. Isotonic recording allows the tissue to contract freely against a constant tension. Isometric recording measures increases in tension of the tissue when the length of the tissue is kept constant. Isotonic recording with smooth muscle probably represents a more physiological type of response than isometric recording, though in the living animal it is probable that all muscles contract partly isometrically and partly isotonically. Isotonic recording tends to produce steep dose-response curves, and this is desirable for bioassay by making the preparation more discriminating. The isometric recording method allows the tissue to remain at an almost constant position on its length-tension relationship, and relaxation of tension is relatively rapid.

Table 1. Physiological salt solutions (Ringer solutions) (salts in g/5 litre).

	Tyrode	De Jalons	Ringer Locke	Frog Ringer	Krebs	McEwens
NaCl	40.0	45.0	45.0	32.5	34.5	38.0
NaHCO$_3$	5.0	2.5	1.0	1.0	10.5	10.5
D Glucose	5.0	2.5	5.0	—	10.0	10.0
KH$_2$PO$_4$	0.25	—	—	—	0.8	—
NaH$_2$PO$_4$	—	—	—	—	—	0.72
KCl	1.0	2.1	2.1	0.7	1.8	2.1
MgSO$_4$.7H$_2$O	—	—	—	—	—	—
MgCl$_2$	0.5	—	—	—	1.45	—
Sucrose	—	—	—	—	—	22.5
CaCl$_2$.2H$_2$O *or* (ml/5l of M solution)	1.32 (18 ml)	0.4 (2.7 ml)	1.6 (10.9 ml)	0.79 (5.4 ml)	1.85 (12.7 ml)	1.5 (10.1 ml)
Aeration	air	95% O$_2$/5% CO$_2$	O$_2$	air	95% O$_2$/5% CO$_2$	95% O$_2$/5% CO$_2$

Notes to Table 1

This table has been compiled from many sources including formulae used in several pharmacology departments in London. The disparity which exists between these teaching institutions is truly remarkable. The greatest differences relate to the calcium concentration; for example I have been able to find four different values for calcium chloride in De Jalons solution. Whether the differences are a reflection of transpositional errors throughout the years or are modifications made on academic grounds is not clear. It must be said however that despite the differences in formulations isolated tissue pharmacology is very much alive at all of these departments. The formulae in Table 1 is the best concensus of all my sources of information but the following modifications do appear to be in use and work equally well:

Tyrode
MgSO$_4$.7H$_2$O 0.6 g instead of MgCl$_2$
MgCl$_2$ 1 g
CaCl$_2$.2H$_2$O 1.25 g
De Jalons
CaCl$_2$.2H$_2$O, 0.2, 0.32, 0.38 g
MgCl$_2$ 0.025 g

Ringer Locke
D Glucose 10 g + CaCl$_2$.2H$_2$O 1.5 g
NaHCO$_3$ 2.5 g + CaCl$_2$.2H$_2$O 1.2 g
Frog Ringer
NaCl 30 g + Na HCO$_3$ 0.5 g + KCl 0.38 g + CaCl$_2$.2H$_2$O 0.63 g
Glucose 10 g + NaH$_2$PO$_4$ 0.5 g + KCl 0.14 g + CaCl$_2$.H$_2$O 1 g

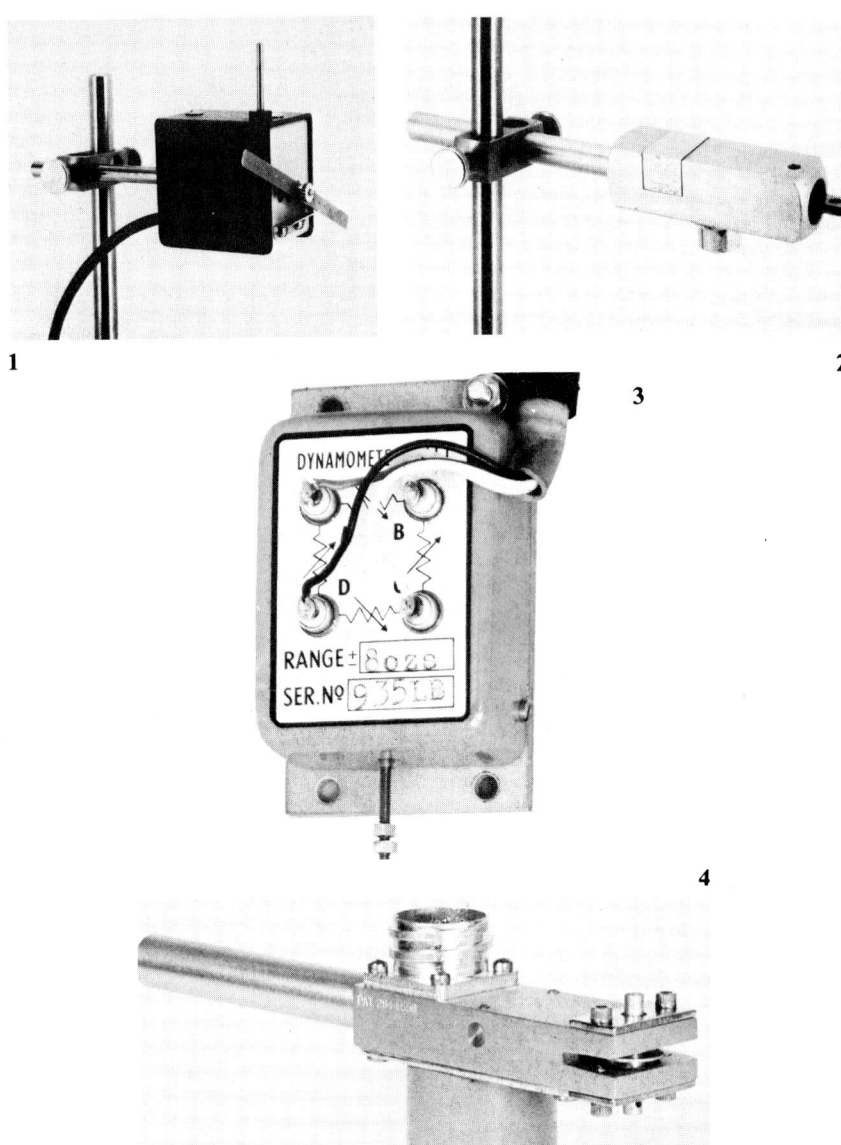

Fig. 2. Pharmacological recording transducers.
1 General purpose isotonic transducer
2 General purpose isometric transducer
3 High sensitivity isometric transducer
4 High sensitivity force displacement transducer for isometric or isotonic measurement
(Photographs provided by Harvard Apparatus (1, 2) Ormed (3) and Grass Instrument Company (4))

Relatively cheap isotonic transducers are available for measurement of length changes. Most designs have their own battery power supply and employ a lever arrangement pivoted on a fulcrum. Movement of the transducer lever is converted into an electrical potential which can be amplified and recorded as a pen movement on a chart recorder trace. Isotonic transducers can be coupled directly into flat-bed potentiometric recorders or into physiological amplifier/recorders. Isometric transducers (force displacement, or resistive strain gauges) usually consist of a cantilever arrangement connected up to four bonded strain gauges which form a fully active Wheatstone bridge network. Force applied to the rigid cantilever mechanisms is transmitted into an output voltage from the bridge circuit. This type of transducer cannot be readily used with a flat bed recorder since it requires an activating voltage to complete the full bridge circuit. It is possible to buy power supplies which serve this purpose, but some pharmacological applications of isometric recording involve fast pen movements which potentiometric recorders are unable to cope with. The more sophisticated pre-amplifier/recorder machines are therefore more desirable for use with isometric transducers. Where pre-amplifier circuitry is not required (e.g. when measuring movements which generate large tensions) bridge coupling units can be substituted, and these are substantially cheaper.

One of the disadvantages of resistive strain gauges is their sensitivity to temperature, and temperature changes will add to the change in resistance induced by mechanical activity. Generally, strain gauges are made of materials whose resistances are highly sensitive to change in dimensions and less sensitive to temperature fluctuations. It is nevertheless important to connect transducers to recording apparatus well in advance of the proposed experiment to ensure temperature equilibration.

2.4 Resting tension and equilibration

Incorrect loading of the tissue is a common error which many students commit. The resting load places the tissue under tension, and it varies for different preparations. Those which are robust and produce powerful contractions in response to drugs are given higher resting tension loads than those which only exhibit small drug-induced tension changes. It is most important that tissues are set up at the recommended resting tension; too much and the tissue will not contract in response to drugs, too little and the resting baseline will be erratic. For isometric recording the bridge of the strain gauge is balanced to the pre-set zero baseline with the resting tension loading weight attached to the transducer. The weight is then removed and replaced by the cotton attached to the tissue. The tension is increased using an adjust-able transducer stand until the recorder pen again reaches the pre-set baseline, thus loading the tissue to the weight originally hung from the transducer. For isotonic transducers, the weight is attached at a point equidistant from the fulcrum and the point of attachment of the tissue. The lever mechanism is then balanced to the horizontal position when the tissue is secured.

The placement of resting tension baseline depends on the response being studied. For those tissues which show contraction only, the baseline is set about 0.5 cm above the lowest point of pen movement. For those tissues which exhibit relaxation only, the baseline is set about 0.5 cm below the maximum upper point of pen movement. The baseline for tissues which respond with contractions and relaxations (e.g. cardiac preparations) should be mid-trace. It is important to ensure that the recorder pens are always kept between the limits of their excursions.

Having been removed from its physiological environment, manipulated in room temperature Ringer and transferred to an organ bath it is only to be expected that preparations require some time before they will respond consis-tently to drugs. An effort should be made to leave tissues for the full equili-bration time, and it is always a golden rule to set up the preparation before making up drugs—a rule which often is not heeded.

2.5 Dose cycle and contact time

The need for regular and consistent methodology in experiments with bio-logical tissues cannot be too highly emphasised. A consistent resting tension, thorough washing and an undisturbed equilibration period should be followed by an experiment which sticks as rigidly as possible to a regular dosing schedule. Biological variation will always mean as much as $\pm 10\%$ in the tissue response. This figure will only be increased if the tissue is treated in an irregular fashion.

The term dose cycle refers to the time between drug additions. Time clocks can be zeroed when the drug is washed out of the bath or when running a baseline. For many preparations the recording of movement is not required continuously. Recorder pen writers should be switched off during dose cycles, but it must be remembered to run a baseline before the next drug addition. It is always tempting to reduce dose cycle times and with very rigid dosing schedules this is possible with some preparations (e.g. guinea-pig ileum). With others, however, (e.g. vas deferens) a reduction in dose cycle often leads to marked tachyphylaxis, i.e. decreased responses to drugs upon repeated dos-ing.

A typical protocol for a dose cycle using guinea-pig ileum is given below:

0 min   Run recorder baseline.
0.5 min   Add drug, observe response.
1.5 min   Switch off recorder, wash preparation.
3 min   Run recorder baseline.

It is more difficult to be precise over drug contact time (i.e. the duration of drug presence in the organ bath) and the figures given in the book should only be used as a guide. The contact time should be chosen from the speed of response of the tissue to a pilot dose. It will be noticed how the speed of response can vary markedly even from tissue removed from the same animal. It is common to base contact times on the time taken to reach a maximal response. Drug contact should not, however, be unnecessarily prolonged as tachyphylaxis can be an associated problem.

2.6 Methods of nerve stimulation

2.6.1 Direct nerve stimulation

If both muscle and its innervating nerve are dissected out of the animal intact it is a simple procedure to attach hook or jaw electrodes to the nerve and then record muscle movements in response to nerve stimulation. This method is employed in Expts. 4.5 and 6.7.

Where the nerve lies alongside a tendon as in the chick biventer cervicis preparation (Expt. 4.7) the tendon is pulled through a ring electrode and current passed through the tendonous tissue to stimulate the nerve. A similar method is employed in the Finkleman preparation (Expt. 2.4). The nerves to be stimulated run periarterially in the mesentery supply to the intestine. The mesentery is pulled through a Saxby ring electrode and the nerve stimulated through the surrounding tissue. This electrode is named after its designer Mr O.B. Saxby (see Burn and Rand, 1960). The various types of electrodes are shown in Fig. 3.

2.6.2 Transmural stimulation

This method was introduced by Paton in 1954 to study the nerve networks of the small intestine, where direct cholinergic nerve stimulation is hampered by insufficient anatomical separation of the pre-synaptic and post-synaptic elements. One electrode is placed in the lumen of a strip of intestine and another into the fluid bathing the intestine. A voltage gradient can be created through the gut wall (hence the term transmural), which is not altered by

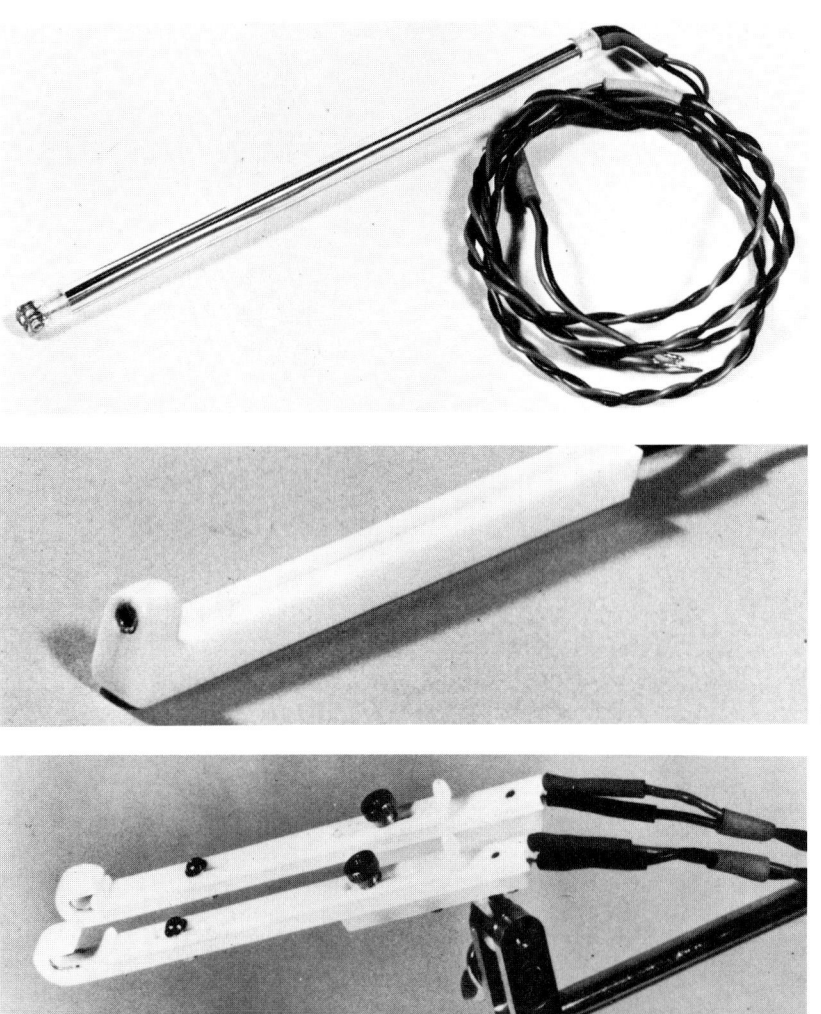

Fig. 3. Types of pharmacological electrode.
1 Saxby electrode for use in, e.g. innervated jejunum preparation
2 Ring electrode for use in, e.g. biventer cervicis preparation
3 Jaw electrode for use in, e.g. perivascular taenia caeci preparation
(Photographs provided by Harvard Apparatus Ltd)

movement of the tissue. The resistance between the electrodes is low and stimulators with a high current output are required. The lumenal electrode should be connected to the positive pole of the stimulator. It is usual to use linear platinum electrodes for transmural stimulation. The intralumenal electrode can, if desired, be welded to a length of fine glass rod which aids passage through the lumen and adds to the rigidity of the electrode. The other electrode should be fixed to the side wall of the organ bath. 0.3–0.5 mm diameter platinum wire is often sufficient for these electrodes.

2.6.3 Field stimulation

An alternative to transmural stimulation, where an internal electrode is sometimes a disadvantage or for some tissues impossible, is field stimulation, where current is passed through the bathing fluid between two external electrodes. High currents are needed for this method since the majority of it is shunted through the physiological salt solution. Measurements of current flow after replacement of tissues by an electrical insulator of similar dimensions indicates that only 0.2% of the applied current passes through the tissue (Harper and Hughes, 1978).

The design of electrodes employed for field stimulation varies considerably. Platinum rings located at the top and bottom of the preparation can be used, or alternatively one ring is sometimes replaced by platinum foil. A third method is to use linear electrodes parallel to the tissue. The differences that such designs produce on neuronally evoked responses have not been fully investigated. Some degree of study has however been made of direct muscle stimulation by field stimulation methods (Speralakis, 1962). The orientation of the electric field has a marked influence on its effectiveness for stimulation. Longitudinal fields (parallel to the longitudinal muscle fibres) are more effective than transverse fields. This may in part be due to differences in tissue reactivities in the transverse and longitudinal directions. The greater resistivity in the transverse directions means that for a given bath voltage gradient, the current density through the tissue (which is of prime concern in stimulation) will be less with a transverse field. These factors may be relevant for neuronally evoked muscle contractions by field stimulation, and therefore longitudinal fields will require lower currents. In connection with this the effect of electrode positions on contractions of guinea-pig isolated ileum to electrical stimulation determines the sensitivity of this preparation to nerve or muscle stimulation. Longitudinal stimulation is least satisfactory for exciting nerves alone (Bennett and Stockley, 1974).

Since large currents are employed using field stimulation heating of the bath must be considered. For a bath of 1 cm² cross sectional area × 5 cm long, and voltage gradient of 10 V/cm, the rise in bath temperature is in the order of 0.5°C/second. Temperature effects will be negligible for field stimulation of neuronal elements since pulse widths are rarely greater than 1 ms.

The dimensions of three typical electrode arrangements are given below.

1 Two linear platinum electrodes (0.3–0.5 mm diameter) are fixed to opposite sides of the organ bath (0.5–1.5 cm apart) so that they run parallel to the tissue. These electrodes should preferably be fused to the glass to ensure a fixed position.

2 Two rings of platinum wire (0.5 mm diameter) are placed at the top and the bottom of the bath. The tissue is located centrally between these rings. The lower ring can be used for attachment of the tissue if a loop of cotton is employed.

3 A coiled platinum wire (0.3 mm diameter) is placed at the bottom of the bath; the second electrode is either a platinum wire projecting 30 mm into the bath or a platinum foil (0.025 mm diameter) ring at the top of the bath.

Field stimulation is sometimes referred to as transmural stimulation; strictly speaking this use is incorrect.

2.7 Stimulus parameters

Details of operation of stimulators is provided in Section 4. Simple 'student' stimulators are sufficient for many applications. Square wave (rectangular) pulses can be delivered at varying frequencies, pulse width and voltage. Nervous stimulation usually requires pulse widths about 1 ms duration or less; direct muscle stimulation requiring larger pulse widths. A characteristic of smooth muscle response to nerve stimulation is frequency dependence. The stimulus intensity simply determines the number of nerves stimulated. Most commercially available stimulators are of constant voltage design, though for many pharmacological applications constant current supplies would be more appropriate. Stimulus intensity is usually expressed as voltage. The term supramaximal is commonly used. It is a little vague and often incorrectly applied. With respect to the experiments described in this book, supramaximal strength is a voltage just greater than that required to produce a maximal response of the tissue.

For field stimulation high output stimulators are required, which often have the facility to deliver trains of pulses. Short trains of high frequency stimulation elicit contractile responses at lower current strengths than single rectangular pulses. Which method is more physiological is a matter of conjecture. A parameter of voltage for field or transmural stimulation intensity has little meaning unless the resistance across the bath is known. Where appropriate, the intensity is expressed as current. Current can be monitored by measuring voltage drop across a series resistor (15Ω). The resistor is placed between the organ bath and the ground side of the output of the stimulator. The voltage drop (V) observed for each stimulus pulse can be converted to current (i) in amps since the resistance (R) is known and i = (V/R). The voltage control on a stimulator can then be preset to deliver a certain current with a specific organ bath and electrode system. Throughout the book voltage parameters are given for field stimulation experiments and these refer to the linear platinum electrode system described in 2.6.3(1). The necessary current intensity is provided in parentheses.

Simple constant current generators can be built and connected to basic stimulators, which provide the pulse width and frequency of stimulation. The

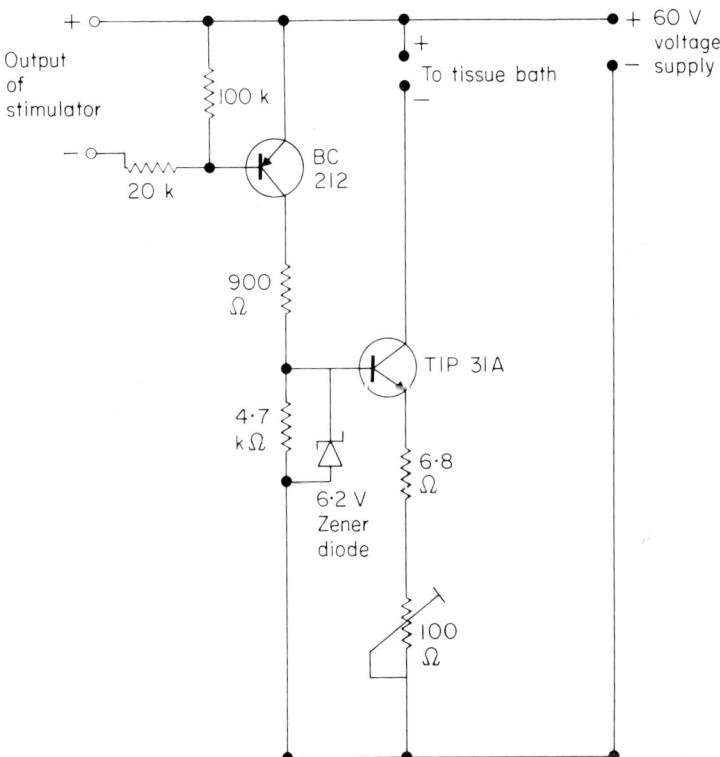

Fig. 4. Constant current generator (designed by Mr Tom Going, Chelsea College, University of London).

limit of current output is dependent on the voltage supply used to power the constant current device. A circuit diagram of a constant current generator is given in Fig. 4. Using a 60 V supply across a typical field stimulation organ bath (2.6.3) currents up to 800 mA can be applied across the bath.

3 Operation of recording apparatus

At the beginning of a course in practical pharmacology a lot of time is often wasted, not only because the student is unfamiliar with the 'knobs and buttons' on the recording apparatus but also, and perhaps more importantly, the student fails to understand the simple electronic principles that govern the workings of the recorder. The precise layout and variety of controls vary from manufacturer to manufacturer but the basic controls are essentially common, and their function is described below. At the present time, there are three types of pharmacological recorders which differ in their degree of sophistication: the flat bed potentiometric recorder, the intermediate medium gain direct writing oscillograph, and the high gain preamplifier/recorder (polygraph).

3.1 Flat-bed potentiometric recorder

3.1.1 Applications

1 All isotonic transducer recording except where tissue movement is extremely small (< 0.5 cm).
2 Isometric recording (if a separate power supply is used to provide an excitation voltage) except where the tension generated by the tissue is small (< 1 g) or the response of the tissue is extremely rapid (full scale deflection of most flat-beds takes 400 ms: field stimulated response of mouse vas deferens peaks at 250 ms).

3.1.2 Controls and functions

1 *Pen zero.* A rotary potentiometer is used to set the recorder baseline.
2 *Coarse gain.* A rotary switch or a series of pushbuttons are used to select the sensitivity of the recorder to the transducer output. It is usually calibrated in mV which refers to the input requirement from the transducer that will produce a full scale deflection of the recorder pen. Alternatively calibration

in mV/cm refers to the input voltage required to produce a 1 cm deflection.

3 *Variable (fine) gain.* Some (but by no means all) flat-bed recorders have a variable gain potentiometer which allows fine adjustment of the sensitivity between each coarse gain setting. Mostly these controls are not calibrated and the variation is usually between 40% and 100% of the coarse gain setting selected.

4 *Polarity switch.* Some flat-bed recorders have polarity switches which determine the direction of pen movement in response to transducer movement. For those flat-bed recorders without this facility, pen movement in the opposite direction to that desired can be simply corrected by reversing the positive and negative input leads.

5 *Chart speed.* A rotary switch or a series of pushbuttons are used to control the speed of the chart trace. Several speeds in either mm/sec or mm/min are usually available.

6 *Event marker.* Occasionally an event marker pen is provided so the trace can be marked when drug additions are made.

3.2 Intermediate (medium gain) direct writing oscillograph

3.2.1 Applications

1 All isotonic transducer recording except where tissue movement is extremely small (< 0.5 cm).

2 Isometric recording (if a strain gauge facility coupler is used) except where the tension generated by the tissue is small (< 1 g). These recorders are suitable for recording rapid twitch responses as the rise time for attaining full scale deflection is < 20 ms.

3 Pressure recording (if a strain gauge facility coupler is used).

4 Integrated rate recording (if a rate facility coupler is used in conjunction with a strain gauge).

3.2.2 Controls and functions

These recorders are supplied with interchangeable plug-in facility couplers which are connected through a main driver amplifier. The functions on each coupler are described below.

Driver amplifier

1 *Pen zero.* A rotary potentiometer is used to set the recorder baseline.

2 *Coarse gain.* A rotary switch (attenuator control) is used to select the sensitivity of the recorder to the transducer output. It is usually calibrated in mV/cm which refers to the input voltage required to produce a 1 cm deflection.

Strain gauge coupler

1 *Balance control.* A rotary multi-turn potentiometer is used to balance the transducer circuit to the zero baseline, which is pre-set with the coupler in the 'off' position.

2 *Polarity switch.* Some couplers have polarity switches which determine the direction of pen movement in response to transducer movement.

3 *Variable gain control.* Some couplers have the facility of a variable sensitivity adjustment which can be used in conjunction with the coarse gain control.

Rate coupler

1 *Range control.* Two or more switched ranges allow the recorder to be set for a full scale deflection.

2 *Trigger control.* A rotary potentiometer is used to ensure that the signal to be integrated triggers the rate meter correctly.

Chart speeds and event markers are supplied as described in 3.1(5) and (6). In addition a time marker in seconds or minutes is usually available.

3.3 High gain pre-amplifier recorder (polygraph)

3.3.1 Applications

1 All isotonic transducer recording (modifications may be necessary to some transducers as not all are compatible with the pre-amplifier inputs or are more appropriately used with the driver amplifier).

2 All isometric recording.

3 All pressure recording.

4 Integrated rate recording (if a tachograph pre-amplifier is used in conjunction with a high gain D.C. pre-amplifier).

3.3.2 Controls and functions

Most pre-amplifier/recorders employ interchangeable plug-in units. Most have separate driver amplifier and pre-amplifiers which can be used separately if required. There is usually a set of inputs for the driver amplifier as well as the pre-amplifier and when the output of the transducer is high (e.g.

isotonic) the high amplification afforded by the pre-amplifier is not required. The functions of the driver and pre-amplifiers and tachographs are described below:

Driver amplifier

1 *Pen zero.* A rotary potentiometer is used to set the recorder baseline. To use this control in isolation (as is required when setting the baseline) a zero switch must be selected. This is sometimes located on the pre-amplifier rather than the driver amplifier.

2 *Driver sensitivity.* A rotary switch or potentiometer (sometimes calibrated in mV/cm) is provided where the driver amplifier is used alone. When the pre-amplifier is used a specific setting on this control may be selected.

Pre-amplifier

1 *Input selector.* Some pre-amplifiers have a variety of input facilities. For most applications described in this book only the full bridge input is required. Some pre-amplifiers have an additional zero setting mode where the input to the pre-amplifier is short circuited. A rotary potentiometer (often a screwdriver control) is used to balance the pen to the pre-set baseline before connecting the transducer in line.

2 *Coarse gain.* A rotary switch (sometimes referred to as 'range' or 'sensitivity' control) is used to select the sensitivity of the recorder to transducer output. It is usually calibrated in mV/cm.

3 *Fine gain.* A rotary potentiometer provides variable sensitivity between about 40% and 110% of the range selected.

4 *Coarse and fine balance.* Two controls are used to balance the transducer to the pre-set zero bascline. The coarse balance is either a rotary switch or a screwdriver control variable potentiometer. This is initially used to roughly balance the transducer. The fine (back-off) control provides precise balancing and this rotary potentiometer can usually be locked. The balancing procedure should be completed on the highest sensitivity setting expected to be used during the experiment.

5 *High frequency filters.* A variable filter (damping) control is usually provided. Sometimes it is located on the driver amplifier. Calibration is sometimes in arbitrary units or in Hz, and refers to damping (usually about 3dB top cut) at that frequency. This control is used to fileter out high frequency vibration picked up by the transducer when the pre-amplifier is used at high sensitivity settings. It is important that the minimal degree of filtering is used to provide a steady baseline. Check that the filter setting used does not attenuate the response of the tissue. For example, the response of the mouse vas deferens to field stimulation is so rapid that filtering of > 5 Hz reduces the twitch height obtained.

6 *Calibration switches.* Many pre-amplifiers and driver amplifiers are adorned with calibration switches. It is worth noting that the majority are irrelevant to the use of amplifiers for measuring isolated tissue movements. The reason for this is that muscle response is expressed in units of mg or g tension generated by the muscle. Therefore to calibrate traces weights can be hung from the transducer and pen movements noted at various sensitivity settings. Thus, as long as sensitivity control settings have been noted during the experiment the recorder pen movement can be expressed in terms of generation of tension. Driver amplifiers and pre-amplifiers usually have calibration buttons which when depressed provide a specified voltage across the input. The variable sensitivity setting can be set for a specific pen deflection but it is mostly unnecessary. One exception is the use of pressure transducers calibrated for the amplifier used. A calibration switch corresponding to 100 mm Hg is useful to pre-calibrate a trace and should be employed when a quantitative assessment of pressure changes is required.

7 *Miscellaneous controls.* One or two additional controls which appear on amplifiers are worthy of mention. A 50 Hz frequency filter is sometimes available to remove mains borne interference. Polarity switches on balance controls allow the direction of pen movement to be changed. In addition a range selector switch on the balance control varies the degree of pen movement per movement of the balance potentiometer.

Tachograph

The tachograph times the interval between peaks or troughs of an AC input (e.g. contractions and relaxations) from a pre-set trigger point and instantaneously integrates a rate from this information (Fig. 5).

1 *Trigger controls.* Several switches control the input derived from the amplifier recording an alternating input. A common set of switches is described below:

A voltage input switch set according to the output from the pre-amplifier.

A slope switch which determines the triggering position of the tachograph either on the leading edge (beginning) or trailing edge (ending) of the pulse.

A rotary threshold switch to determine the precise point of triggering on the waveform. It should be set as close to the maximal peaks and troughs of the input that provides a constant triggering. This position will provide the most accurate integration of rate.

2 *Calibration controls.* Before operation the tachograph requires calibration. Usually a switched control in conjunction with a rotary potentiometer

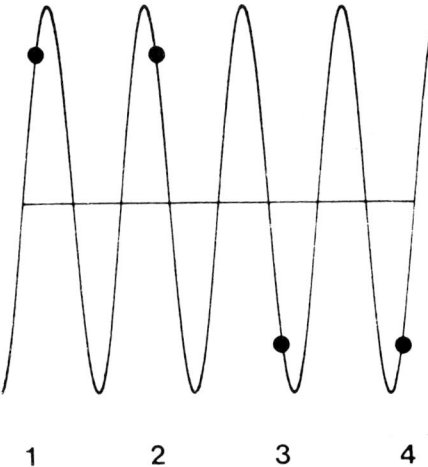

Fig. 5. Trigger points on a.c. input to tachograph.
Possible points for triggering tachograph amplifier:
1 upper pulse, leading edge
2 upper pulse, trailing edge
3 lower pulse, leading edge
4 lower pulse, trailing edge
●The trigger point should be chosen as the most reliably constant point of the a.c. trace.

is used to set a designated pen movement. The tachograph scale (controlled by a rotary switch) is then set. The scale is calibrated in ranges and the limits (expressed in beats/minute) refer to the baseline and full scale deflection calibration. The use mode often has two positions for slow and fast alternating signals and is set accordingly.

Chart speeds and event markers are supplied as described in 3.1.2(5) and (6). In addition a time marker in seconds or minutes is usually available.

3.4. Chart recorder speed

Many students perform experiments perfectly well but finish up with a ragged chart trace of their isolated tissue responses. A neat trace is something which is very easy to achieve and gives a good impression in practical write-ups. Two mistakes lead to poor traces. Firstly, a chart speed that is too fast is a common fault and when the chart is left on between doses it results in an unnecessarily long chart trace which makes comparison of responses less easy. For many experiments described in this book a speed of 5 mm/min will suffice. If responses are unusually fast or slow this may need to be modified accordingly. Secondly, and most importantly, the chart trace should be switched off and the pens removed from contact with the chart paper when the tissue is washed. The rules for neat traces are as follows:

1   Run a baseline (0.5 cm) before drug additions.

2   When maximal response is obtained, switch off chart trace *before* washing and set input switch at zero, so that the pen returns perpendicularly to the baseline.

3   Leave chart switched off until the beginning of the next dose cycle.

4   For field stimulated responses run intermittently, when maximal response is obtained remove pens from the trace *before* washing, and then set input switch to zero. Run the trace on 1 cm before beginning next dose cycle and start stimulator before replacing pens on the trace as the first stimulus sometimes produces large artifact responses.

5   For traces run continuously, for example, some field stimulated preparations or preparations producing a continual myogenic response, momentarily remove the pens from the chart trace during washing.

4 Operation of pharmacological stimulators

Operation of pharmacological stimulators may pose problems similar to those encountered with the electronic recording apparatus. The following section is intended to help familiarise the student with the controls and functions found on stimulators and also to explain the simple electronic principles behind the type of stimulus provided. For the experiments described three types of pharmacological stimulator may be used: 1, basic square-wave (student) stimulator; 2, dual pulse square wave stimulator; 3, advanced multi-function square-wave stimulator (Fig. 6). The functions available from each stimulator are shown diagrammatically in Fig. 7.

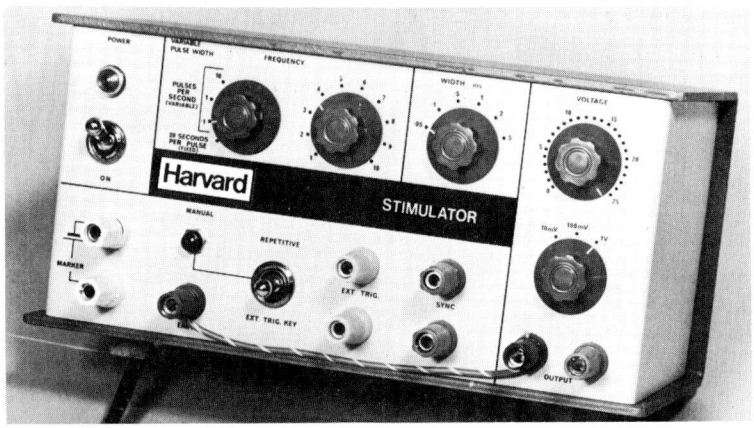

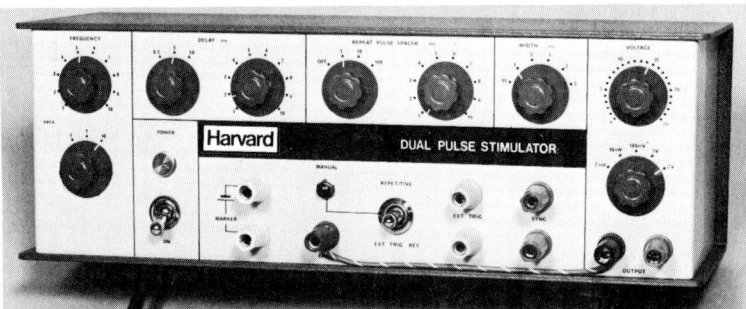

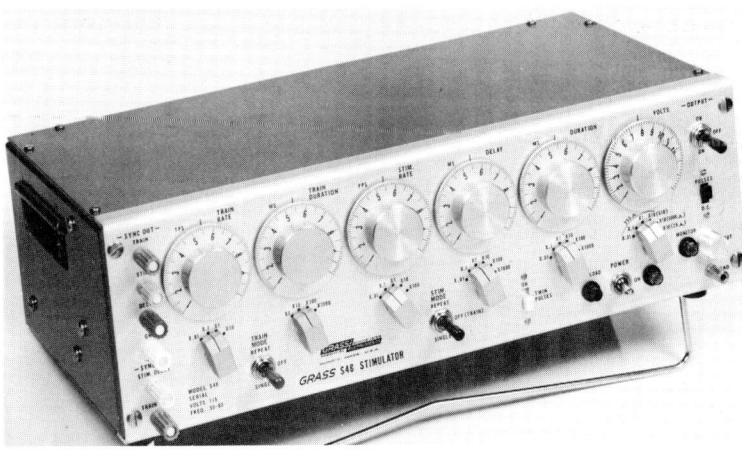

Fig. 6. Pharmacological stimulators.
1 Basic square-wave stimulator
2 Dual pulse square-wave stimulator
3 Advanced multi-function square-wave stimulator
(Photographs provided by Harvard Apparatus Ltd. (1, 2) and Grass Instrument Company (3)

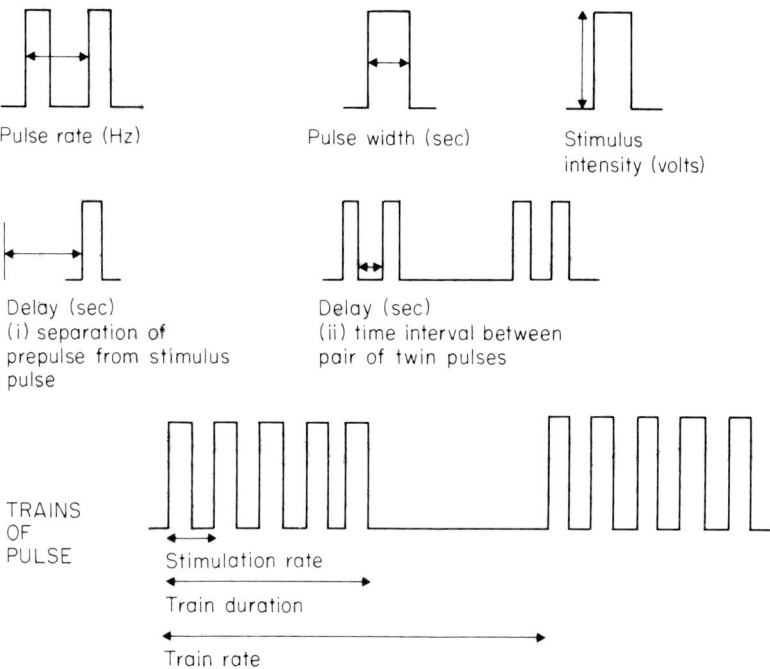

Fig. 7. Stimulator functions.

4.1 Basic square-wave stimulator

4.1.1 Applications

All experiments employing direct nerve stimulation.

4.1.2 Controls and functions

1 *Pulse switch.* Up to three positions are provided. One position provides continuous repetitive pulses (at the frequency selected). The second position provides a single pulse usually operated manually by a pushbutton or a spring toggle switch. The third position can be used for external triggering via a pair of terminals.

2 *Pulse width.* A rotary switch provides variations in the duration of the rectangular pulses from about 0.05 ms–5 ms.

3 *Frequency.* Usually a rotary switch and a single-turn potentiometer control the number of pulses delivered per second and the settings on each control are usually multiplied to give the frequency in Hertz (Hz). Variation between 0.1 and 100 Hz are common.

4 *Stimulus strength (amplitude).* Usually a rotary switch and a single-turn potentiometer control the amplitude of the pulse and the settings on each control are usually multiplied to give the strength in volts. Up to 25 V is normally available.

4.2 Dual pulse square-wave stimulator

4.2.1 Applications

All experiments employing direct nerve stimulation and transmural stimulation. Field stimulation can also be provided if the stimulator is of the high output type (i.e. up to 150 V).

4.2.2 Controls and functions

1 *Pulse switch.* As 4.1(1) except that in addition dual (twin) pulses can be provided.

2 *Pulse width.* As 4.1(2) except employing a rotary switch and a single-turn potentiometer control allowing variation from 0.01–100 ms.

3 *Frequency.* As 4.1(3) except variable from 0.1–1000 Hz.

4 *Stimulus strength (amplitude).* As 4.1(4) except variable up to 150 V for some stimulators.

5 *Delay.* A rotary switch and a single-turn potentiometer control the delay circuit time. This control allows a delay between a synchronising pulse from an external source and an output pulse allowing an oscilloscope to be pre-triggered. No experiments in this book utilise this switch. The delay is usually calibrated from 0.1–100 ms.

6 *Dual pulse spacer.* In the dual pulse mode the delay between the two pulses is determined by two variable controls as for frequency, delay or pulse width. The spacer is usually variable from 1–100 ms. On some stimulators this control is designated as a delay control. It can function as in (5) and sets the time interval for the twin pulse pair.

4.3 Advanced multi-function square-wave stimulator

4.3.1 Applications

All experiments employing direct nerve, transmural and field stimulation (including trains of pulses stimulation).

4.3.2 Controls and functions

1 *Pulse switch.* As 4.1(1) including dual (twin) pulse switch plus additional switch for operation in trains of pulses mode.

2 *Pulse width (duration).* As 4.1(2) allowing variation from 0.01 ms–10 s.

3 *Frequency (rate).* As 4.1 (3) allowing variation from 0.01–1000 Hz.

4 *Stimulus strength (voltage).* As 4.1(4) allowing variation from 15 mV–150 V. Outputs up to a maximum of 400 mA are often available.

5 *Delay.* As 4.2(5) allowing variation from 0.01 ms–10 s. Commonly in the twin pulses mode this control determines the interval between pulses, as in 4.2(6).

6 *Train rate.* A rotary switch and a single-turn potentiometer control the rate at which trains of pulses are delivered; variable from 0.01–1000 trains per second. Therefore in the train mode this control is identical to the frequency control (3). The frequency control is then set to determine how many pulses occur within the set train duration (see 7).

7 *Train duration.* A rotary switch and a single-turn potentiometer control the length of time a train of pulses, of a given rate, delay and strength are delivered. Variable from 1 ms–10 s.

5 Drug preparation, storage and concentrations

Many drugs are made up in concentrated stock solutions and diluted for the experiment. Final dilutions should be made with the physiological salt solution used in the experiment or 0.9% saline. Where very small volumes are added in relation to bath size it may be permissible to add drug dissolved in distilled water. The storage of drugs varies enormously and is often dependent on the concentration and pH of the stock solution. Storage at $+4°C$ is recommended to discourage the growth of micro-organisms and storage at $-25°C$ is necessary for some compounds. Details of special precautions for the storage of some drugs is given in Table 2. Addition of ascorbate should be restricted to a concentration of 20 μg/ml since it can affect drug-induced responses at higher concentrations.

The experimental parameters section for each group of experiments is followed by a list of drug concentrations for use in the experiments. They should be used as a guide only, and it must be appreciated that the variation in sensitivity of biological tissue to drugs can be quite large. It should also be noted that chosen concentrations of antagonists should be tailored to the sensitivity of the tissues to agonists. If agonist concentrations used are much less than recommended, antagonist concentrations should be reduced proportionally. The data given throughout the book refer to final bath concentrations to be used as starting doses. Dose response curves should be carried out by using two-fold stepwise increases in dose from this original starting concentration. When alternative concentrations are employed these are included in the text of each individual experiment.

Volumes of drug addition should not exceed 10% of the total bath volume, and strictly speaking concentrations should be expressed in molarity which makes it unnecessary to specify the salt of the drug used. It is still a common practice to use concentrations in weight/volume (e.g. mg/ml), and w/v concentrations will be given throughout. These concentrations relate to the commonly used salts of the drugs which are given in Table 2. It is important to understand how to convert to molarity and definitions of some terms relating to concentration are given below:

Molar solution (M)	The molecular weight of a substance dissolved in 1 litre of water.
Mole	Molecular weight of a substance in grams
mg (milligrams)	10^{-3} of a gram
μg (micrograms)	10^{-6} of a gram
ng (nanograms)	10^{-9} of a gram
pg (picograms)	10^{-12} of a gram
fg (femtograms)	10^{-15} of a gram

Table 2. Molecular weights and storage of commonly used salts of drugs

Drug salt	M.W. of salt	M.W. of base	Comments
Acetylcholine chloride	181.7	146.2	Unstable in dilute aqueous solutions
Adrenaline bitartrate	333.3	183.2	Unstable: add ascorbate
Amethocaine hydrochloride	300.8	264.3	
Angiotensin amide	—	1031.2	
Atropine sulphate (anh)	676.8	289.4	Salt contains 2 molecules of base
Barium chloride	208.3	—	
Bradykinin	—	1060.3	Unstable: store on ice
Bretylium tosylate	414.4	243.2	
Bromolysergic acid diethylamide	—	402.4	
Carbachol chloride	182.7	147.2	
Cimetidine hydrochloride	288.5	252.0	
Clonidine hydrochloride	266.6	230.1	
Cocaine hydrochloride	339.8	303.4	

Table 2. Molecular weights and storage of commonly used salts of drugs—*contd.*

Drug salt	M.W. of salt	M.W. of base	Comments
(D-Ala², D-Leu⁵)-enkephalin acetate	629.7	569.7	Use fresh: plastic containers
Dexamphetamine sulphate	368.5	321.8	
Diphenhydramine hydrochloride	291.8	255.4	
Dopamine hydrochloride	189.7	153.2	Unstable: add ascorbate
Ephedrine hydrochloride	201.7	165.2	
Ergometrine maleate	441.5	325.4	
Guanethidine sulphate	494.7	198.3	Salt contains 2 molecules of base
Hexamethonium bromide	362.2	256.3	
Histamine dihydrogen phosphate	307.1	111.2	Salt contains 2 molecules of base
5-hydroxytryptamine creatinine sulphate	387.4	176.2	
Indomethacin	—	357.8	Insoluble in water: Dissolve in polyethylene glycol or EtOH
Iproniazid	—	179.2	
Isoprenaline hydrochloride	247.7	211.2	Unstable: add ascorbate
Leucine—enkephalin acetate	615.8	555.7	Use fresh: plastic containers
Mepyramine maleate	401.5	285.4	
Methacholine chloride	195.7	160.2	
Methionine—enkephalin acetate	633.7	573.8	Use fresh: plastic containers
Methysergide hydrogen maleate	469.5	353.5	
Morphine sulphate	668.8	285.3	Salt contains 2 molecules of base
Naloxone hydrochloride	363.9	327.4	
Neostigmine bromide	303.2	267.7	
Nicotine	—	162.2	
Noradrenaline bitartrate	337.3	169.2	Unstable add ascorbate
Oxytocin	—	1007.2	
Papaverine hydrochloride	375.8	339.4	Insoluble in water: sparingly soluble in EtOH
Phenoxybenzamine hydrochloride	340.3	303.8	Sparingly soluble in water: dissolve in EtOH and add an equal amount of 0.1 M HCl
Phentolamine mesylate	377.5	281.4	
Phenylephrine hydrochloride	203.7	167.2	
Physostigmine salicylate	413.5	275.3	Unstable: add ascorbate
Practolol	—	266.3	

Table 2. Molecular weights and storage of commonly used salts of drugs—*contd.*

Drug salt	M.W. of salt	M.W. of base	Comments
Procaine hydrochloride	272.8	236.3	
Propranolol hydrochloride	295.7	259.3	
Prostaglandin E_1	—	354.5	Unstable: store on ice
Prostaglandin $F_2\alpha$	—	368.5	Unstable: store on ice
Salbutamol sulphate	288.4	239.3	
Sodium cromoglycate	—	512.3	
Sodium nitrite	69.0	—	
Suxamethonium chloride. $2H_2O$	397.3	290.3	Unstable: use fresh
Tetrodotoxin	—	319.3	
Thymoxamine hydrochloride	315.8	279.3	
Tryptamine hydrochloride	196.7	160.2	
(+)-tubocurarine chloride. $5H_2O$	771.7	610.0	
Tyramine hydrochloride	173.6	137.2	
Vasopressin	—	1005.0	
Yohimbine hydrochloride	390.9	354.4	

6 Measuring responses

Most of the experiments described are based on the ability of isolated tissues to produce dose-related responses to added drugs. For many preparations quantitation is simple. For example, guinea-pig ileum produces a contraction in response to acetylcholine which is maximal after about 30 seconds. The height of contraction is measured from the steady baseline to the top of the drug-induced response. The response is usually expressed as a percentage of maximum if achieved, and plotted against log dose. Not all tissues, however, have a steady baseline. Some exhibit spontaneous activity and the mid-point of these movements must be taken for measurement of any drug-induced effect. Others (e.g. frog rectus) show a rising baseline due to increased muscle tone, and the movement of the tissue due to this must be taken into account when measuring drug-induced responses. Quantitation of inhibitory effects on very marked spontaneous activity (e.g. Finkleman preparation, Expt. 2.4) can be achieved by measuring the area of inhibition. This method takes into account the absolute reduction in muscle contraction, the duration of inhibition and the time for recovery after washing.

Increasing use is being made of drug-induced inhibition of field or transmurally stimulated muscle twitch responses. Whether a preparation is stimulated continually or only prior to drug administration, constant twitch reponses are aimed for. The drug is usually left in contact with the tissue until a maximal inhibitory effect is attained. Percentage inhibition is then expressed as:

$$100 - \left(\frac{\text{Twitch response at maximal inhibition} \times 100}{\text{Control twitch response immediately prior to drug addition}} \right)$$

When the twitch responses lack consistency a mean of control and maximally inhibited contractions can be taken. In such circumstances however, it is often better to discard the tissue in question. Inhibitory dose values (ID's) can either be related to the absolute inhibition or to the percentage of maximum inhibition. In some tissue where 100% inhibition is attainable these two estimates will be identical. Thus an ID_{50} value will be expressed as either the dose required to produce a 50% inhibition or the dose required to produce an inhibition which is 50% of the maximum attainable inhibitory response.

The majority of experiments described employ dose responses achieved by intermittent dosing of the tissue on a fixed dose cycle. In some preparations the tissues may be very slow to recover from dosing or may be markedly disrupted by washing. The preferred method of measuring dose responses in these instances is by cumulative dosing. Maximal effect is achieved for each drug dose before a subsequent incremental dose is added to the organ bath without washing. A full cumulative dose response curve is therefore achieved at each dosing interval.

For the purpose of making cumulative dose response curves it is important that the bath volume is not too small and the added drug volumes should be kept to a minimum. The total added volume of drug should not exceed 5% of organ bath volume.

For a number of tissues, dose response curves made in the conventional way and cumulative dose response curves are virtually identical. However, cumulative dosing has not proved as popular as the conventional and more time consuming method, and seems only to be resorted to when methodological conditions dictate the need. Cumulative dosing itself poses certain methodological problems. For example, when using isometric recording, contractile responses may fade with some agonist drugs and isotonic measurements are best in these circumstances. In addition, drugs which are broken down by enzymes in the organ bath also exhibit fading of responses and only stable compounds are really suitable for cumulative dosing studies. Furthermore, single doses are less likely to lead to tachyphylaxis and for some drugs this phenomenon is prominent.

7 Fault finding

There is nothing more frustating in pharmacology practicals, than to spend considerable time setting up a preparation only to find it does not respond to drugs or, where appropriate, electrical stimulation. However, many students waste considerable time persevering or dithering with isolated tissues without really knowing where to begin investigating what could be wrong. Students could equally argue that lecturing or demonstrating staff are sometimes at sea in sorting out problems. When in doubt, the Krebs Ringer is often used as a scapegoat!

There should be no need to waste time on isolated tissues that do not appear to work. A systematic approach to fault finding can very quickly determine if the preparation is potentially viable or if another preparation needs to be attempted. If after correcting a fault the tissue is still unsatisfactory don't waste time 'persevering', it will invariably lead to disappointing results. Instead set up another tissue if possible.

A great deal of fault finding sounds very obvious but there is an extra-ordinarily broad spectrum in a student's ability to diagnose what is wrong, just as there is for locating breakdown faults in vehicles. The following section is intended as a guide to quick diagnosis, and is set out in a similar fashion to how you would find it in a car handbook.

Symptom	Possible fault	Corrective measure
A. Recording system failure (recorder pen does not respond to manual operation of transducer)	1. Recorder pen failure	Check for pen movement with recorder zero.
	2. Amplifier failure	Check for increased pen movement by increasing amplifier gain. Check if bridge is balanced.
	3. Transducer failure	Check battery (isotonic only)
B. Tissue does not respond (drugs or stimulation)	1. Recording system failure	See A
	2. Too much resting tension	Rebalance transducer
	3. Bath temperature too low	Check temperature of inner organ bath
	4. Ringer solution faulty	Replace Ringer
	5. Electrode failure and faulty drug solutions	Check electrode and replace drug solutions
C. Tissue responds to agonist but does not show dose-related responses	1. Too much resting tension	Rebalance transducer
	2. Bottom or top of dose reponse curve	Increase or decrease dose fourfold

Symptom	*Possible fault*	*Corrective measure*
	3. Insensitive to agonist—flat dose response relationship	Investigate activity of another agonist
D. Tissue shows reduced responses to agonist drugs after repeated dosing	1. Tachyphylaxis (drug tolerance *in vitro*)	Increase dose cycle
E. Tissue responses are graded but show only small pen movements on recorder	1. Amplifier gain too low	Increase amplifier gain sensitivity
	2. Baseline set below lower limit of pen excursion	Rebalance amplifier to ensure that baseline is above lower limit of pen excursion
	3. Transducer (isotonic) lever set on lower limit of movement (fulcrum rest)	Raise transducer so that lever is free to move
F. Tissue responses are graded but pen movements are maximum on trace	1. Amplifier gain too high	Decrease amplifier gain sensitivity
	2. Transducer (isotonic) lever movement reaches maximum limit (fulcrum rest)	Reattach tissue at a point closer to the fulcrum and rebalance *or* reduce size of tissue
G. Tissue shows movement but pen recorder does not respond	1. Recording system failure	See A
	2. Transducer bridge not balanced	Rebalance transducer
	3. Transducer (isotonic) lever fixed on lower or upper limits of movement	Balance lever to a central position
H. Tissue contracts when located in organ bath and remains contracted after repeated washing	1. Ringer solution contains agonists or impurities from previous experiments	Replace Ringer in reservoir
	2. Ringer solution faulty	Replace Ringer
I. Baseline rises and stimulated response (where appropriate) is not constant	1. Insufficient tension (normally due to transducer drift)	Rebalance transducer
	2. Insufficient washing	Increase wash period

Symptom	Possible fault	Corrective measure
J. Baseline falls	1. Too much tension (normally due to transducer drift)	Rebalance transducer
	2. High amplifier gain showing tissue and transducer drift	Reduce sensitivity if possible
K. Baseline irregular and stimulated responses (where appropriate) not constant	1. Insufficient tension	Rebalance transducer
	2. Spontaneous activity of muscle	Increase tension and/or decrease bath temperature. Regular drug dosing sometimes improves spontaneous activity
L. Variable responses for equal drug concentrations administered in different volumes	1. Volume artifacts (usually observed with small organ baths)	Use constant volumes
	2. Insufficient mixing	Increase aeration
	3. Tissue exposed to bolus of drug by injection directed at tissue	Inject drug away from tissue
M. Tissue does not respond to direct nerve stimulation	1. Recording system failure	See A
	2. Tissue set up failure	See B
	3. Stimulator failure	Check pulse monitor light
	4. Insufficient voltage	Increase stimulator voltage output
	5. Portion of nerve not viable	Move electrode closer to nerve/muscle junction
	6. Electrode failure	Replace electrode
	7. Nerve not viable	Replace preparation
N. Tissue does not respond to field stimulation	1. Recording system failure	See A
	2. Tissue set up failure	See B
	3. Stimulator failure	Check pulse monitor light
	4. Electrode failure	Check for bubble formation on positive electrode in response to repetitive pulses at high outputs
	5. Preparation not viable	Try increasing resting tension: replace tissue
O. Field stimulated response initially poor but improves with time	1. Insufficient washing	Wash tissue with Ringer until response improves
	2. Initial exposure to H_2O present in aeration line	Always prime apparatus with Ringer with aeration line fully open

Symptom	*Possible fault*	*Corrective measure*
	3. Insufficient equilibration period	Allow longer before beginning stimulation
	4. Insufficient initial resting tension	Increase tension during equilibration period
P. Field stimulated response initially good but deteriorates with time	1. Insufficient tension (normally due to transducer drift)	Rebalance transducer
	2. Stimulator output current/voltage too high	Reduce output or stimulate intermittently
	3. Insufficient washing between drug additions	Increase washing and/or dose cycle
	4. Repeated exposure to cold Ringer	Ensure volume used for washing does not exceed warming coil volume
Q. Tissue responds to direct nerve stimulation but response deteriorates with time	1. Polarity incorrectly connected	Reverse polarity
	2. Too high stimulator output	Reduce voltage
R. Stimulated responses preceeded by downward pen movement on trace	1. Stimulation artifact	Move transducer or transducer leads away from electrode leads: reverse polarity
S. Krebs ringer solution goes cloudy in organ bath	1. CO_2 not being supplied in aeration line	Replace Ringer in bath and ensure O_2/CO_2 aeration

Isolated Uterus

Introduction

The uterus is innervated by sympathetic nerves and possibly a parasympathetic supply which runs to the wall of the tissue. The response of the uterus to drugs varies from species to species, the uterus of the rabbit gives responses which closely approximate those of the human. In contractile response this tissue is atypical of smooth muscle. There is often a latent period after drug addition before initiation of contraction, the response is invariably all or none, and the contracture is not maintained even when the drug is still present. This failure to sustain contraction is a physiological phenomenon known as transient depolarisation. An all or none response or a very steep log dose response curve is often observed with cholinergic agonists. The dose response characteristics of the tissue are temperature and Ringer dependent, and steep dose response curves are obtained at 37°C. 32°C is usually chosen for experiments with the uterus in order to reduce spontaneous contraction. Such activity is also reduced by using a low Ca^{++} Ringer such as De Jalons solution, and inducing oestrus in the animal by prior injection of an oestrogen. Uterine responses to drugs may also vary throughout the oestrus cycle.

It seems likely that uterine muscle contracts mainly isometrically, and isometric recording is to be favoured. In addition, when using an isotonic transducer, investigation of drug effect on uterine muscle is sometimes difficult, especially with rabbit muscle, because the tissue contracts rhythmically, but in an irregular fashion and the responses to drugs tend to be all or none. Using an isometric transducer, however, minimises spontaneous contractions and can often produce graded drug responses.

Drugs

Cholinergic agonists. Drugs which stimulate muscarinic receptors such as acetylcholine, carbachol and methacholine all produce contraction of the uterus.

33

Adrenoceptor agonists. The relative proportions of α- and β-adrenoceptors, mediating contraction and relaxation respectively varies from species to species and between oestrus and dioestrus. In the rat, β-receptor responses remain constant but α-receptors appear under the action of oestrogen. The β-receptor response predominates, but it is sometimes preceded by a transient α-receptor mediated contraction for mixed α- and β-agonists. Since the isolated uterus has no inherent tone, relaxation can only be observed by physiological antagonism of the contractile responses to drugs such as acetylcholine. Adrenaline is about 100 times more potent in producing relaxation of rat uterus than noradrenaline. This relative difference in potency was once used for assaying adrenaline contaminated with noradrenaline. The rat uterus is a good example of a tissue containing β-adrenoceptors and β-receptor mediated relaxation of this preparation can be blocked with β-receptor antagonists such as propranolol.

Indirectly acting sympathomimetics. Both tyramine and ephedrine are not very active on this preparation since their primary mode of action is to release noradrenaline from sympathetic nerve terminals. Ephedrine is slightly more effective probably by virtue of its direct agonist activity at α- and β-adrenoceptors.

Oxytocin and vasopressin. Oxytocin has a high selective action on the smooth muscle of the uterus, and stimulates both electrical and contractile activity. The sensitivity of the uterus to oxytocin is slight except at full term. Vasopressin stimulates the uterus when it is least sensitive to oxytocin. Thus, the non-pregnant human uterus, and the uterus in early pregnancy are more sensitive to vasopressin than to oxytocin.

Ergometrine. Ergometrine is by far the most potent alkaloid of ergot in causing uterine contractions, but it does not possess adrenoceptor blocking activity. Contraction of the uterus becomes forceful and prolonged and resting tone is markedly increased. The degree of sensitivity of the uterus to ergometrine varies with the degree of maturity.

Barium ions. Barium stimulates all muscle and is highly toxic. By virtue of its action on uterine muscle, it may, like other heavy metal ions, cause abortion in pregnancy.

Autacoids. Smooth muscle of the rat is particularly insensitive to the actions of histamine and uterine muscle is no exception. 5-Hydroxytryptamine on the other hand often produces dose-related contractions of the uterus. The receptors which mediate this response are of the so-called D type (p. 42) and antagonised by methysergide.

Uterine smooth muscle responds to prostaglandins, though the responses are very dependent on the state of the uterus. $PGF_{2\alpha}$ causes contraction of the non-pregnant uterus and PGE_2 relaxation. It is also possible that generation of prostaglandins within this smooth muscle contributes to the response to some agonists. This possibility is investigated in Expt. 1.3.

Experimental parameters

Organ bath		20 ml
Ringer solution	Rat	De Jalons
	Rabbit	Krebs
Aeration		95% O_2/5% CO_2
Bath temperature	Rat	32°C
	Rabbit	37°C
Recording	Rat	Isotonic
	Rabbit	Isometric
Resting tension	Rat	0.5 g
	Rabbit	1 g
Equilibration period		30 minutes
Dose cycle		3 minutes
Contact time		15–30 seconds

Drugs (final bath concentration: starting dose)

	Rat	Rabbit
Acetylcholine	50 ng/ml	500 ng/ml
Adrenaline	100 ng/ml	100 ng/ml
Atropine	100 ng/ml	250 ng/ml
Barium chloride		250 μg/ml
Carbachol	100 ng/ml	
Ephedrine	50 μg/ml	
Ergometrine		5 μg/ml
Histamine	500 μg/ml	
5-Hydroxytryptamine	10 ng/ml	
Indomethacin	5 μg/ml	
Isoprenaline	10 ng/ml	10 ng/ml
Methysergide	1 ng/ml	
Noradrenaline	1 μg/ml	100 ng/ml

Oxytocin		0.01 U/ml
Phentolamine	10 ng/ml	
Physostigmine		250 ng/ml
Propranolol	10 ng/ml	
Prostaglandin $F_{2\alpha}$	20 ng/ml	
Tyramine	50 μg/ml	
Vasopressin		0.01 U/ml

Expt. 1.1 Cholinergic and adrenergic drugs and the rat uterus

The preparation is based on the method of De Jalon et al. (1945). Inject a female rat with 0.1 mg/kg stilboestrol intramuscularly 24 hours before the experiment. Kill the rat by dislocating the neck and exsanguinate the animal. Open the abdomen and expose the two uterine horns by pulling aside the intestine. They are often easily distinguishable by their pink colouration. Uterine smooth muscle is very sensitive to stretching and great care must be taken not to subject it to undue tension. Free each horn from surrounding fat and mesenteric attachments, cut each horn out separately, and transfer them

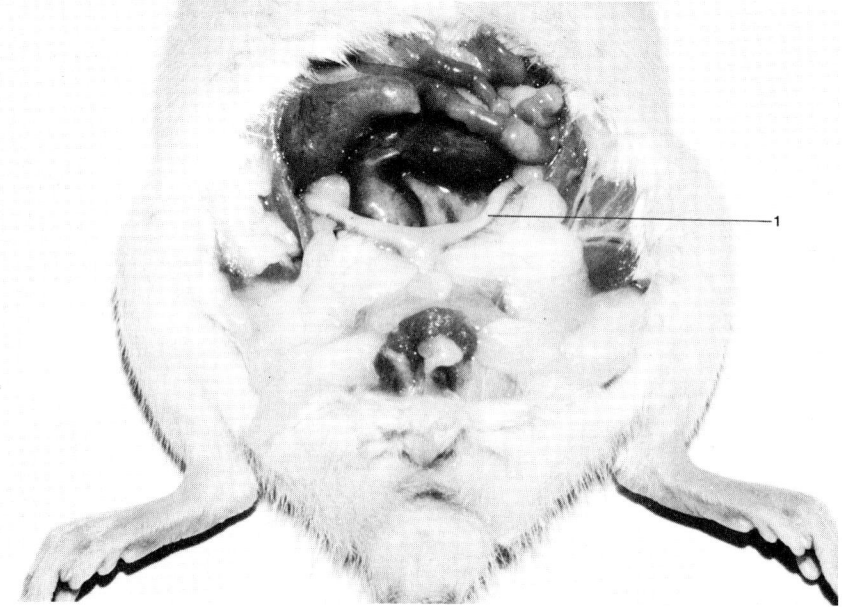

Fig. 8. Dissection of rat uterus. The uterine horns (1) are exposed and removed from the animal.

to a petri dish containing De Jalons Ringer. Depending on the size of the uterus the two horns can be further divided, by making a transverse cut, into four preparations (3–4 cms each). The tissue will work quite adequately as a tube, but longitudinal cuts can be made and the tissue set up as a sheet of muscle if preferred.

Pass threads through one wall of the uterus at both top and bottom. Attach the bottom thread to the tissue holder, transfer it to an isolated organ bath and attach the top thread to the transducer.

Experimental protocol

1 Show responses of the uterus to acetylcholine and carbachol, and investigate whether these responses are all or none.

2 Add adrenaline and leave in contact with the tissue for one minute, followed without washing by a standard acetylcholine dose. Attempt to show a 50% reduction in the acetylcholine response. Repeat acetylcholine doses until the response returns to the control level.

3 Repeat 2 for noradrenaline.

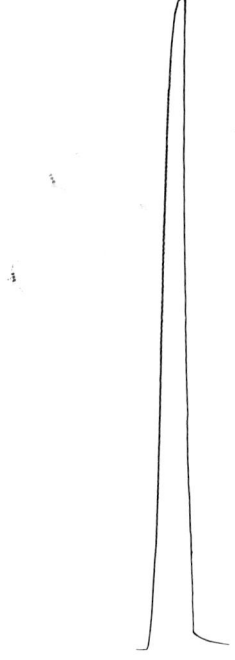

Fig. 9. Response of the rat uterus to acetylcholine (▲ 1 μg/ml).

4 Repeat 2 for isoprenaline.

5 Repeat 2 for tyramine.

6 Repeat 2 for ephedrine.

7 Add phentolamine and leave in contact for 5 minutes. Repeat 2 and 3 maintaining the phentolamine concentration in the bath.

8 Add propranolol and leave in contact for 5 minutes. Repeat 2 and 3 maintaining both phentolamine and propranolol concentrations in the bath.

This experiment should show the response of the uterus to cholinergic agonists and the physiological antagonism of these responses by adrenaline, and at higher concentrations, noradrenaline. The relative lack of effect of indirectly acting sympathomimetics is investigated and the receptors mediating the adrenaline/noradrenaline antagonism is also elucidated.

Expt. 1.2 5-Hydroxytryptamine, histamine and the rat uterus

Set up the uterus as described in Expt. 1.1.

Experimental protocol

1 Show responses of the rat uterus to 5-hydroxytryptamine and construct a dose response curve if possible.

2 Show the insensitivity of this preparation to histamine.

3 Add atropine to the bath and leave in contact for 10 minutes. Repeat a submaximal dose of 5-hydroxytryptamine. Increase the atropine concentration fivefold and repeat the 5-hydroxytryptamine.

4 Add methysergide to the bath and leave in contact for 10 minutes. Repeat the dose of 5-hydroxytryptamine chosen in 3. Increase the dose of methysergide to show abolition of 5-hydroxytryptamine responses.

The lack of effect of atropine on 5-hydroxytryptamine responses is shown in this experiment, which contrasts with the results obtained with similar concentration of atropine on guinea-pig ileum (Expt. 2.2). In contrast a selective D-receptor antagonist (p. 42), methysergide, abolishes 5-hydroxytryptamine responses.

Expt. 1.3 Responses of the rat uterus to agonists after inhibition of prostaglandin synthesis

Set up the uterus as described in Expt. 1.1.

Experimental protocol

1 Show dose related responses to oxytocin, prostaglandin $F_{2\alpha}$ and acetylcholine.

2 Add indomethacin to the Ringer reservoir and equilibrate for 20 minutes.

3 Repeat (i).

Indomethacin which inhibits prostaglandin sythesis should antagonise oxytocin induced contractions but have little effect on responses to acetylcholine and protaglandin $F_{2\alpha}$ suggesting that endogenous prostaglandins may contribute to the stimulant activity of oxytocin.

Expt. 1.4 Drugs and the rabbit uterus

Set up the uterus as described for the rat in Expt. 1.1.

Experimental protocol

1 Investigate the effects of noradrenaline and adrenaline at the same concentrations.

2 Show responses to acetylcholine.

3 Add isoprenaline to the bath and leave in contact for 2 minutes and then without washing repeat a submaximal acetylcholine dose. Repeat acetylcholine responses until they return to their control level.

4 Repeat 3 for physostigmine (3 mins).

5 Repeat 3 for atropine (3 mins).

6 Add oxytocin and observe the response.

7 Add vasopressin and observe the response.

8 Repeat the noradrenaline dose used in 1.

9 Add ergometrine and leave in contact for 10 minutes and then withou washing repeat 8.

10 Show the effect of barium chloride.

This experiment should show the physiological antagonism of acetyl- choline responses by isoprenaline and pharmacological antagonism anc potentiation of acetylcholine responses by atropine and physostigmine re- spectively. The uterine stimulant activity of oxytocin, vasopressin, ergometrine and barium ions is also studied. Ergometrine should have no effect on the α-mediated responses of noradrenaline.

Isolated Small Intestine
(Qualitative experiments)

Introduction

Intestinal muscle is innervated by both parasympathetic and sympathetic fibres of the autonomic nervous system. The parasympathetic fibres synapse at two ganglionic sites, in the myenteric (Auerbachs) plexus and in the submucous (Meissners) plexus. The myenteric plexus lies between the longitudinal and circular muscle coats, the longitudinal fibres being present on the outer surface of the intestine. Most experiments involve the investigation of drug action on the contractions of the longitudinal muscle. Sympathetic fibres also innervate the intestine, and usually run periarterially through the mesentery to the muscle. Peristaltic movements are myogenic and mainly initiated by local reflexes. This peristaltic reflex can occur without any neural connections to the brain or spinal cord, and the extrinsic nerves to the intestine appear to have only a minor role in modulating the activity of the organ. Stimulation of sympathetic nerves inhibits peristaltic movements, whilst parasympathetic stimulation increases peristaltic activity. The parasympathetic action is mediated via muscarinic receptors, whilst the inhibitory effects of sympathetic stimulation are mediated via α- and β-adrenoceptors. Thus the intestine is unusual in that both α- and β-receptor types mediate a similar biological response. The β-receptors are probably of the β_1-type, and it has been suggested that they are located on smooth muscle fibres, whilst the inhibitory α-adrenoceptors are located presynaptically on parasympathetic ganglion cells of the myenteric plexus.

The myogenic, spontaneous activity of the intestine varies along its length and from species to species. The caecal end of the guinea-pig ileum, for instance, gives a steady baseline which is important for studying drug-induced contractions. The caecal end is unusual however as α-adrenoceptors mediate excitatory responses. Spontaneous activity is often artificially reduced by running the experiment at a temperature some 5–7°C below normal body temperature. Rat, mouse and rabbit intestine exhibit spontaneous activity. This strong and consistent response of rabbit intestine is used for the study of relaxation produced by sympathetic nerve stimulation or sympathomimetic drugs.

40

Stimulation of sympathetic nerves to rabbit jejunum may be achieved by periarterial stimulation, a method described by Finkleman (1930) (Expt. 2.4). If the preparation is very fresh, and taken from a young rabbit it is sometimes possible to observe parasympathetic effects by using low stimulation rates (2–4 Hz). Higher rates of stimulation produce exclusively sympathetic effects, and the effects of drugs on adrenergic transmission can accordingly be studied.

Stimulation of the intramural nerves of the guinea-pig ileum can be achieved by either using transmural or field stimulation (see pp. 9 and 11). The nerve plexus in the wall of the gut is complex and has been described as providing a paradigm of mechanisms at synapses in the central nervous system. The myenteric plexus-longitudinal muscle strip is a very useful alternative preparation when field stimulation is employed. The main benefits of this preparation are that the tissue is much less complex. In the studies of ACh, for instance, one only needs to consider Auerbachs plexus. In addition muscle spasm is reduced since circular fibres are absent, and the onset and offset of drug action is more rapid.

Different parts of the small intestine are used in pharmacological experiments. In man, the small intestine is sub-divided into a duodenum, which is short and devoid of mesentery, a jejunum which accounts for the proximal two-fifths of the remainder of the intestine, and an ileum which accounts for some three-fifths of the organ. These proportions show small variations from species to species. The duodenum of the mouse and rat, for instance, is only a few millimetres long.

Drugs

Cholinergic agonists and antagonists. Drugs which stimulate muscarinic receptors cause contraction of the isolated intestine and their effects can be blocked by appropriate antagonists such as atropine. Contractions can also be induced by stimulation of parasympathetic ganglia with nicotinic agonists, which causes the postganglionic neurone to fire and this results in the release of acetylcholine at the neuroeffector cell junction. These effects can therefore be antagonised by muscarinic antagonists as well as ganglion blockers such as hexamethonium. The actions of nicotine are complex and it is often a difficult drug to work with. Tachyphylaxis to the contractile effects of nicotine is common and high doses will block ganglionic transmission.

Autacoids. Histamine and 5-hydroxytryptamine both contract intestinal muscle and these effects can be blocked by H_1-antagonists, such as mepyramine, and 5-hydroxtryptamine antagonists respectively. The receptors which mediate the 5-hydroxytryptamine response were originally designated M and D (Gaddum and Picarelli, 1957), from their original studies which showed that morphine and dibenzyline (phenoxybenzamine) alone could partially block 5-hydroxytryptamine induced contractions. A mixture of both morphine and dibenzyline completely antagonised 5-hydroxytryptamine responses. This hypothesis has not gone uncriticised but there has been relatively little attention paid to peripheral 5-hydroxytryptamine receptors in recent years. The terminology is a little confusing since it is now standard to use methysergide or bromolysergic acid diethylamide (BOL) as a D-receptor antagonist and atropine or phenylbiguanide as an M-receptor antagonist. In addition the D-mediated response results from a direct stimulant action on the smooth muscle whilst the M-mediated response is associated with nervous elements within the intestine. The latter response appears to be due to stimulation of ganglion cells causing the postganglionic neurones to release acetylcholine. Tryptamine also stimulates the isolated intestine, an effect mediated by D-receptors since contractions are completely blocked by methysergide. It is becoming apparent that there are several types of 5-hydroxytryptamine receptors and those in the central nervous system appear to be distinct from those in the periphery in terms of their susceptibility to antagonists.

Adrenergic agonists. Sympathomimetic drugs have a predominantly inhibitory action on the intestine. This effect is only observed as a relaxation in intestinal muscle which has spontaneous activity, such as the rabbit jejunum. Guinea-pig ileum on the other hand has no inherent tone *in vitro* and the inhibitory effect of adrenergic agonists can only be observed by showing physiological antagonism of a contractile response elicited by, for example, histamine or acetylcholine.

Adrenergic blocking drugs. The inhibitory effects of mixed α- and β-receptor agonists can be blocked by mixtures of phentolamine and propanolol. The inhibitory effect of sympathetic nerve stimulation in the rabbit Finkleman preparation can be blocked by adrenergic neurone blocking drugs (ANB's) such as guanethidine and bretylium whilst the sensitivity to exogenously applied receptor agonists is retained. The effects of ANB's can be reversed by some indirectly acting sympathomimetics e.g. dexamphetamine. Uptake blockers such as imipramine also antagonise the adrenergic neurone blocking activity of bretylium, but are without effect against guanethidine if adrenergic neurone block is established.

Opioids. Morphine inhibits the release of acetylcholine from cholinergic nerves and contractile responses induced by stimulation of intramural cholinergic nerves can be blocked by morphine. Whilst the effects of opioids on the guinea-pig intestine are mediated predominantly by μ-opioid receptors mouse ileum contains predominantly δ-opioid receptors and the enkephalins are very active at inhibiting the stimulated response in this preparation.

Experimental parameters

Organ bath	Mouse ileum (transmural stimulation)	5 ml
	Guinea-pig ileum	20 ml
	Guinea-pig ileum (field stimulation)	10 ml
	Rabbit jejunum	30 ml
	Rabbit jejunum (periarterial stimulation)	50 ml
Ringer solution	Unstimulated intestine	Tyrode
	Stimulated intestine	Krebs
Aeration	Tyrodes	Air
	Krebs	95% O_2 5% CO_2
Bath temperature	Mouse	30°C
	Guinea-pig	32°C
	Rabbit	37°C
Recording	Guinea-pig and rabbit	Isotonic
	Stimulated Guinea Pig and Mouse	Isometric
Resting tension	Mouse	0.2 g
	Guinea-pig	0.5 g
	Rabbit	0.5–4 g
Equilibration period		30 minutes
Dose cycle	Mouse	see Expt. 2.6
	Guinea-pig	2–3 minutes
	Rabbit	3–5 minutes
Contact time	Mouse	see Expt. 2.6
	Guinea-pig	15–30 seconds
	Rabbit	30 seconds
Stimulus parameters:	Expt. 2.4 Pulse width	1 ms
	Voltage	Supramaximal
	Frequency	1–50 Hz
	Stimulus duration	30 s

Expt. 2.5	Pulse width	0.5 ms
	Voltage	20 V (150 mA)
	Frequency	0.1 Hz
Expt. 2.6	Double Pulse	
	Pulse width	1 ms
	Pulse spacer	40 ms
	Voltage	20 V (> 50 mA)
	Frequency	0.3–0.5 Hz
Expt. 2.7	Double pulse	
	Pulse width	1 ms
	Pulse spacer	50 ms
	Voltage	40 V (150 mA)
	Frequency	0.05 Hz

Drugs (final bath concentration: starting dose)

	Guinea-pig	Rabbit	Mouse
Acetylcholine	5 ng/ml	10 ng/ml	
Adrenaline	50 ng/ml	5 ng/ml	
Atropine	1 ng/ml	1 ng/ml	
Bretylium		1 μg/ml	
Carbachol		10 ng/ml	
Dexamphetamine		20 μg/ml	
Diphenhydramine	1 ng/ml		
Ephedrine		10 μg/ml	
Guanethidine		1 μg/ml	
Hexamethonium	1 μg/ml	1 μg/ml	
Histamine	5 ng/ml	100 ng/ml	
5-Hydroxytryptamine	50 ng/ml		
Isoprenaline		5 ng/ml	
Leucine enkephalin	300 ng/ml		1 ng/ml
Methionine enkephalin			1 ng/ml
Morphine	2 ng/ml		100 ng/ml
Naloxone	100 ng/ml		100 ng/ml
Nicotine	1 μg/ml	1 μg/ml	
Noradrenaline	50 ng/ml	5 ng/ml	
Phentolamine		500 ng/ml	
Phenoxybenzamine	50 ng/ml		
Physostigmine		100 ng/ml	
Propanolol		500 ng/ml	
Tetrodotoxin	1 μg/ml		
Tyramine		10 μg/ml	

Expt. 2.1 Agonists and antagonists on the guinea-pig ileum

The preparation is based on the method of Magnus (1904). Kill a guinea-pig
by dislocating the neck and exsanguinate the animal. Open the abdomen and
expose the caecum. The ileum runs into the central part of the caecum whilst
the large intestine begins from the distal end of caecum. Remove the ileum
from the caecal end and cut into isolated segments (4 cm in length). The
spontaneous activity normally increases the closer the tissue is to the stomach.
Transfer the ileum to a petri dish containing Tyrodes solution and trim away
the mesentery and fat surrounding the muscle. Ileum will remain viable for
several hours in room temperature ringer if aerated. For long periods before
use the tissue can be kept in ringer solution at 4°C. Ideally, the animal should
be starved for 24 hours before killing. If food is present in the ileum it can be
expelled by gently passing Tyrodes solution at 37°C through the lumen by
means of a 5 ml pipette. Pass threads through one wall of the ileum at both
top and bottom and attach the bottom thread to the tissue holder. Transfer
the mounted tissue to the organ bath and attach it to the transducer.

Experimental protocol

1   Show dose-related contractions of the ileum to acetylcholine, histamine
and nicotine.
2   Add adrenaline or noradrenaline and leave in contact with the tissue for
one minute followed without washing by a submaximal dose of acetylcholine.
Repeat acetylcholine until the response returns to the control level.

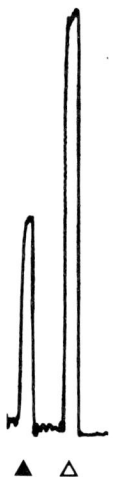

▲ △

Fig. 10. Responses of the guinea-pig ileum
to acetylcholine (▲10 ng/ml, △20 ng/ml).

3   Repeat 2 for histamine instead of acetylcholine after first ensuring that the control response is still present.

4   Repeat 3 for nicotine.

5   Repeat 2 using hexamethonium instead of adrenaline or noradrenaline against acetylcholine.

6   Repeat 5 against histamine, after first ensuring that the control response is still present.

7   Repeat 5 against nicotine after first ensuring that the control response is still present.

8   Add atropine to the bath and leave in contact with the tissue for 2 minutes followed by the submaximal acetylcholine dose. After washing replace the atropine in the bath for a further 2 minutes and repeat the submaximal histamine dose. Wash the tissue and repeat acetylcholine doses until responses return to the control level.

9   Repeat 8 using diphenhydramine instead of atropine.

This experiment should show that several drugs may cause contraction of isolated intestine, mediating their effects via different mechanisms. The responses of acetylcholine and histamine may be difficult to restore after addition of the more persistent antagonists atropine and diphenhydramine. This experiment also forms the basis of a determination of the pharmacological characteristics of an unknown drug provided to a student (see Expt. 2.3).

Expt. 2.2   Antagonism of 5-hydroxytryptamine responses on the isolated guinea-pig ileum

Set up the ileum as described in Expt. 2.1.

Experimental protocol

1   Determine a dose of 5-hydroxytryptamine which produces a submaximal response large enough to show measurable inhibition by antagonists. It may be necessary to intersperse 5-hydroxytryptamine doses with doses of acetylcholine to prevent 5-hydroxytryptamine tachyphylaxis.

2   Add morphine to the bath and leave in contact with the tissue for 1 minute followed by the 5-hydroxytryptamine dose.

3   Double the concentration of morphine in the bath fluid (1 min) and ensure that the degree of inhibition of 5-hydroxytryptamine response is maximal. Wash the tissue and repeat 5-hydroxytryptamine dose until the response of the tissue returns to the control level.

4 Repeat 2 and 3 using phenoxybenzamine instead of morphine.

5 Repeat 2 using phenoxybenzamine and morphine added to the bath together.

This experiment should show the partial inhibition of 5-hydroxytryptamine responses by both morphine and phenoxybenzamine and the total abolition of the response by a combination of the two antagonists, as was observed by Gaddum and Picarelli (1957).

Expt. 2.3 Determination of the pharmacological properties of an unknown drug using rabbit intestine

Kill a rabbit by dislocating the neck and exsanguinate the animal. Open the abdomen and locate the jejunal area of the intestine. This is the proximal part where the mesenteric supply is profuse. Trim the mesentery away and mount a section of intestine in an organ bath as described for guinea-pig ileum (Expt. 2.1) with the exception that washing is accomplished by overflow since exposure of this tissue to air disrupts spontaneous activity.

Experimental protocol

The following drugs are provided: acetylcholine, carbachol, nicotine, histamine, noradrenaline, atropine, hexamethonium, phentolamine, propranolol, physostigmine, together with a solution of X of unknown concentration.

The student is expected to design the experimental procedure. The following notes may help to approach the problem:

1 Never add the unknown drug first, it may be an irreversible antagonist

2 Obtain control responses to known agonists.

3 Rabbit intestine is insensitive to histamine.

4 Dilute the unknown similarly to your dilutions of known standards.

This experiment aims to provide a phamacological characterisation of an unknown drug, not to name the unknown. The myogenic contractions of the jejunum should be regular. Contractile responses induced by ganglion stimulants, parasympathomimetics or drugs acting directly on the muscle are observed over and above the myogenic movements. Relaxation is produced by sympathomimetics or direct muscle relaxants and when there is some inherent tone in the tissue, muscarinic blockers.

Expt. 2.4 Adrenergic neurone blockers and the innervated rabbit jejunum

The isolated spontaneously contracting rabbit jejunum with autonomic innervation is set up according to the method of Finkleman (1930). Locate the jejunal area of the intestine as described in Expt. 2.3. Select a section of intestine leaving a convenient branch of the mesenteric artery (about 3–4 cms) in the mesentery attached to it. Transfer the tissue to a petri dish containing Krebs or McEwens solution and attach threads to one wall of the tissue at both top and bottom. Tie a third thread to the central cut end of the branch of the mesenteric artery. Attach the bottom thread to the tissue holder, transfer the mounted intestine to the organ bath, and attach the top thread to the transducer. Pass the thread attached to the mesentery through the ring of a Saxby electrode (p. 9) and secure this alongside the intestine. Pull sufficient mesentery gently through the ring to facilitate stimulation of autonomic nerves which run periarterially. The electrical connections to the stimulator should be made so that the cathode is nearest to the muscle.

Experimental protocol

1   Show frequency related inhibition of the pendular movements of the intestine by carrying out a frequency response curve (1, 2, 5, 10, 20, 50 Hz). Do not wash the tissue between stimulation.

2   Show dose related inhibition of intestinal movements by carrying out a dose response curve to noradrenaline. Keep wash out periods to a minimum.

3   Add guanethidine to the Ringer solution and leave the tissue to equilibrate for 5 minutes.

4   Repeat the frequency response curve using the higher frequencies only.

5   Repeat the dose response curve to noradrenaline.

6   Add dexamphetamine to the Ringer solution and leave the tissue to equilibrate for 5 minutes.

7   Repeat 4.

This experiment shows the inhibitory effect of guanethidine on sympathetic nerve stimulation, whilst the sensitivity to agonists acting upon post-synaptic adrenoceptors is retained. The indirectly acting sympathomimetic dexamphetamine should reverse the effects of guanethidine. An alternative ANB for study is bretylium and alternative sympathomimetics, tyramine and ephedrine.

Although this is essentially a qualitative experiment the inhibitory effects

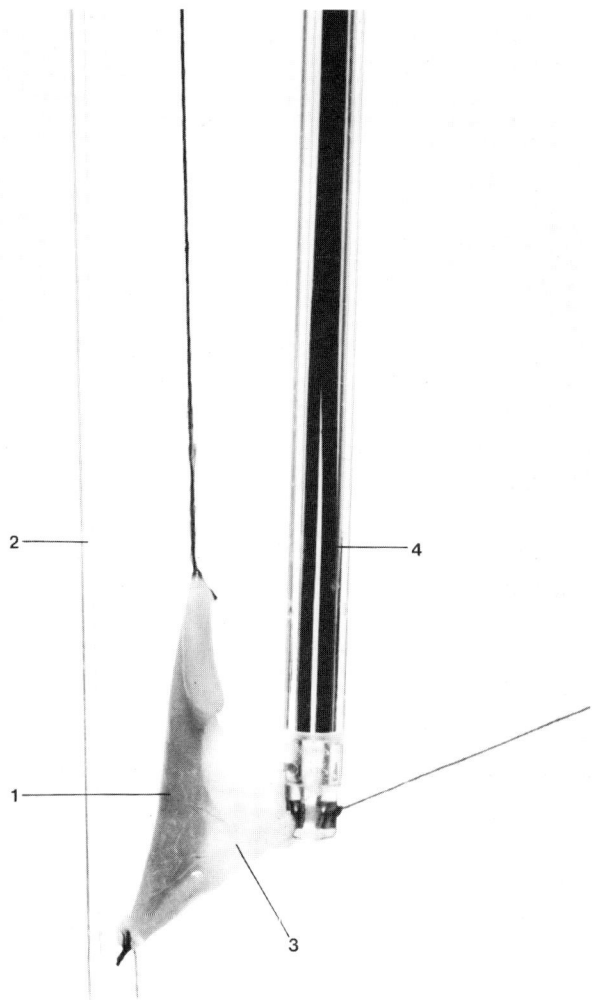

Fig. 11. Innervated rabbit jejunum.

The jejunum (1) is attached to a tissue holder (2) and the upper thread tied to the transducer. The mesentery (3) with the periarterial nerves is pulled through a Saxby electrode (4).

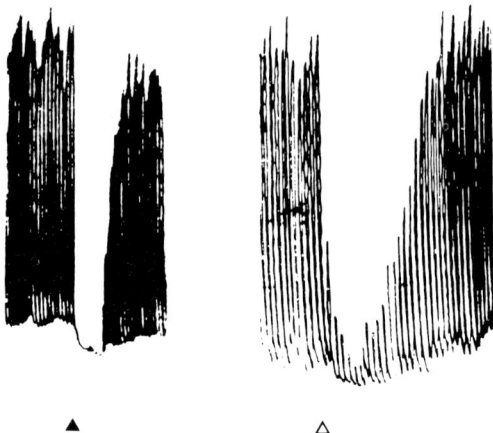

Fig. 12. Responses of the rabbit jejunum to perivascular stimulation (▲ 10 Hz, 30s) and noradrenaline (△ 100 ng/ml).

of stimulation or drugs can be quantified by measurement of the area of inhibition. This area should be traced, then placed on graph paper and the area determined by counting the number of square millimetres.

Expt. 2.5 Field stimulated guinea-pig ileum

Set up a length of guinea-pig ileum as described in Expt. 2.1 in an organ bath with an electrode on either side of it in the bath fluid (see p. 11).

Experimental protocol

1   Show submaximal responses to histamine, acetylcholine and a 3 minute period of field stimulation (0.1 Hz).
2   Show the effect of morphine (100 ng/ml) added to the bath 1 minute after commencing field stimulation.
3   Wash the tissue and repeat 1 plus a stimulation at 50 Hz.
4   Add atropine to the Ringer solution and repeat 1.
5   Raise the concentration of atropine (100 ng/ml) and repeat field stimulation at 50 Hz, and the histamine response.
6   Add tetrodotoxin to the bath and repeat field stimulation and histamine as in 5.
     This experiment provides an indication that neurotransmitters other than

acetylcholine are released from the gut in response to field stimulation. 50 Hz stimulation should be blocked by tetrodotoxin indicating a nerve-mediated response but unaffected by muscarinic blockade, as is 0.1 Hz stimulation. Morphine is used as an example of a drug which inhibits acetylcholine release. Potentiation of exogenous acetylcholine may be observed and is probably due to inhibition of acetylcholinesterase by morphine. The direct effect of histamine upon the intestinal muscle should be retained throughout the experiment.

Expt. 2.6 Transmurally stimulated mouse ileum preparation and opioid drugs

The preparation is based on the methods of Holman and Hughes (1965) and Handa et al. (1981). Remove a length of ileum (3 cm) as described for the guinea-pig in Expt. 2.1. Pass threads through one wall on the same side of the ileum at both top and bottom. Make a loop at one end for attachment to the tissue holder and transfer the ileum to the organ bath. Pass an internal electrode for transmural stimulation (see p. 9) through the lumen of the gut and secure it in place. Attach the top thread to the transducer. After 15 minutes equilibration begin stimulation. A frequency should be chosen to give regular responses on top of the spontaneous rate. This is commonly about 10% greater than the spontaneous rate and 0.3 or 0.4 Hz is usually appropriate. Stimulation should be continued throughout the experiment. Wash the tissue after cumulative dose response curves by overflow.

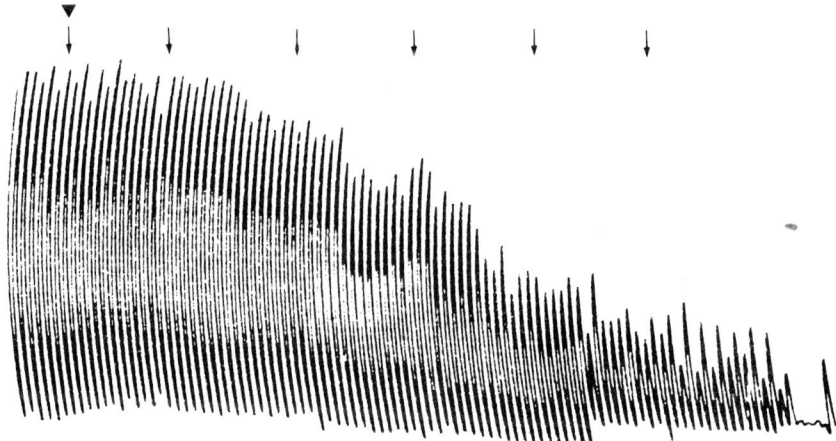

Fig. 13. Responses of the transmurally stimulated mouse ileum to cumulative doses of methionine-enkephalin (▼ 0.2, 0.4, 0.8, 2, 4, 8 ng/ml: 0.4 Hz).

Experimental protocol

1 Carry out cumulative dose response curves (see p. 28) to methionine enkephalin, leucine enkephalin and morphine. Allow a 45-second contact time for each dose and 10 minutes between each drug.

2 Add naloxone to the Ringer solution and leave to equilibrate for 10 minutes.

3 Repeat 1.

Cumulative dose response curves are employed in this preparation since the tissue takes a long time to settle after washing. It is an unusual ileum preparation since it has predominantly δ-opioid receptors and responds well to the enkephalins but is very insensitive to μ-opioid receptor agonists such as morphine.

Expt. 2.7 Field stimulated myenteric plexus-longitudinal muscle strip preparation of the guinea-pig and opioid drugs

The preparation is based on the methods of Rang (1964) and Paton and Zar (1968). Remove a 4–6 cm length of ileum as described in Expt. 2.1 and pull

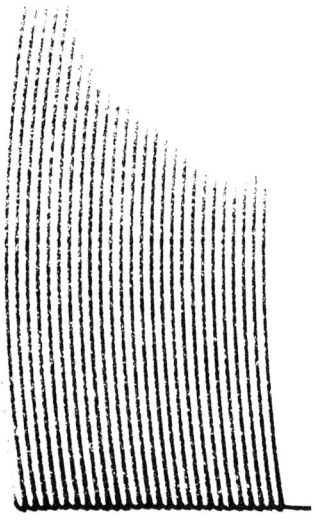

Fig. 14. Response of the field-stimulated myenteric plexus longitudinal muscle strip of the guinea-pig to morphine (▲ 10 ng/ml).

the ileum gently over a glass rod (the tip of a 2 ml pipette is often suitable for this purpose). Locate the point of attachment of the mesentery to the ileal muscle. This is most readily distinguished by the blood vessels which run longitudinally. Take a small piece of cotton wool soaked in Krebs Ringer and carefully stroke the ileal muscle tangentially from the point of mesenteric attachment. As the longitudinal muscle is separated from the underlying circular fibres rotate the glass rod so that the muscle is separated from the total area of ileum present. Transfer the resulting strip preparation to a petri dish and set up (in the longitudinal plane) by tying threads at either end of the muscle and locate in an organ bath designed for field stimulation (see p. 11).

Experimental protocol

1 Carry out dose-response curves to morphine and leucine enkephalin. The preparation can be stimulated continally but if high voltages are used for field stimulation it is best to employ intermittent stimulation and to obtain control responses for 1 minute prior to dosing. Allow 7–10 minutes between drug additions to avoid tachyphylaxis. Maximal inhibitory effects are observed after about 2 minutes.
2 Add naloxone to the Ringer solution and leave to equilibrate for 10 minutes.
3 Repeat 1.

In contrast to the mouse ileum guinea-pig intestinal muscle has a predominantly μ-opioid receptor population. Thus morphine is far more potent than the enkephalins in this preparation and is more readily reversed by the antagonist naloxone which has about a ten-fold higher selectivity for the μ- than for the δ-receptor.

Isolated Small Intestine
(Qualitative experiments)

Introduction

With the development of biochemical and chemical methods for assaying levels of drugs and endogenous substances the use of biological assay has been declining in recent years. Nevertheless, the use of biological tissues for quantitative assessment of agonist and antagonist activity is still very important for our understanding of the mechanisms involved in drug action. For example, recent studies of opioid agonists and antagonists have employed the principle of parallel assay in several peripheral isolated tissues.

Most of the principles of biological assay can be demonstrated using the guinea-pig ileum. The ease with which this preparation can be set up makes it an ideal choice for student practicals.

An example of biological assay (four point) can be found in Expt. 3.1. Measures of agonist potency (pD_2 Expt. 3.3) and agonist affinity constant (Expt. 3.5) can also be determined using the guinea-pig ileum. An example of the bracket assay method is given in Expt. 3.1.

Agonist assays

Four types of biological assay can be employed. All these assays assume that if a response to a dose of 'unknown' is equivalent to the response of a dose of standard then the amount of drug added to the preparation is identical. This assumption presumes that the biological response to the unknown is due only to the drug under investigation and therefore the dose response curves of unknown and standard are parallel.

1 Match assays

This is probably the simplest form of biological assay. It has no place in research, and has severe limitations. It involves matching a response produced by a dose of unknown as closely as possible to a response produced by a known concentration of standard. The responses must be submaximal. The degree of accuracy of this type of assay is markedly dependent on the steepness of the dose response curve. Flat log dose response curves give poor discrimi-

54

nation, i.e. large differences in log dose give only small differences in response. In addition an exact match of response would be difficult to achieve.

2 Single-point log-dose response assays

Single-point assays still have a place in research work and where the tissue response is regular and the dosage regime firmly regulated, reliable results can be obtained. A full dose response curve is constructed for the standard and then unknown solutions are given in volumes which produce submaximal responses. The responses are converted to concentrations by reading directly off the drawn log dose response curve. Greater accuracy can be achieved if a regression line (usually taken from points between 20% and 80% of maximum) is calculated and unknown concentrations calculated from a regression formula (see below). The greater the number of unknowns studied, the greater is the chance of error, as the responses are increasingly further from the original standard doses. Where more than six unknowns are to be determined it is often best to repeat the dose response curve.

Linear regression analysis of log-dose response curves for single-point assays

Formula for a straight line:

$$y = \bar{y} + b(x - \bar{x})$$

where b = slope of the line
$\bar{y}$ = mean of responses
$\bar{x}$ = mean of log dose

and $b = \dfrac{\sum XY}{\sum X^2}$

and $\sum XY = \sum xy - \dfrac{\sum x . \sum y}{N}$

and $\sum X^2 = \sum x^2 - \dfrac{(\sum x)^2}{N}$

N is equal to the number of points included in the line and x represents values of log dose and y values for the tissue response.

For determination of concentration of unknown, substitute response y into formula for a straight line. Values of b, $\bar{y}$ and $\bar{x}$ are known and the corresponding value of x (unknown concentration) can be calculated.

3 Three point assays (bracket and 2 × 1 assays)

The three point assay brings a degree of refinement and therefore greater accuracy to a single-point assay. The simplest type is a bracket assay, and this is still a commonly used method in pharmacological research. Each response produced by a dose of unknown is bracketed either side with responses to doses of standard. The doses of standard are chosen to give one response less than the unknown and the other greater than the unknown. All responses must fall in the linear region of the log dose response curve, and the greatest accuracy can be achieved when the limits of the bracket produced by the standard are close.

e.g. Solution	1 × Standard	Unknown	1.5 × Standard
Response (% of max)	30	40	50

The concentration of unknown can be determined graphically by plotting response against log dose and constructing a line between the two standard points. The responses produced by the unknown can then be converted to a standard concentration.

To minimise error introduced by biological variation a 2 × 1 assay can be employed where the two doses of standard and dose of unknown are given repeatedly and a mean response for each is obtained. It is usual to repeat each standard and unknown four times in a random order. The concentration of unknown can be determined graphically as for the bracket assay or mathematically, e.g.

$$U = \text{antilog} \ \frac{\log (b/a).(z - y) + \log b.(y - x)}{y - x}$$

where a and b = concentrations of agonist used for bracket
         x and y = responses to a and b respectively
             z = response to unknown
             U = concentration of unknown.

4   Four point assays (2 × 2 assays)

This method confers the greatest accuracy in biological estimation of an unknown. It is little used for research purposes as it is extremely time consuming. Two doses of unknown and two of standard are used, thus making four points. Therefore two estimates of the slope of the linear portion of the log dose response curve are obtained, which should be parallel. The order of the four doses of drug are randomised using latin squares and a mean of responses produced by each solution determined. An example of a latin square is:

$$
\begin{array}{cccc}
A & B & C & D \\
B & C & D & A \\
C & D & A & B \\
D & A & B & C \\
\end{array}
$$

This method minimises error due to biological variation and the effect of a previous dose on a subsequent one.

If a and b are the two dose volumes of standard and c and d the two dose volumes of unknown the dose volume ratio of $a:b$ must equal the dose ratio of $c:d$, e.g. if a and b are 0.1 and 0.2 ml respectively and c is 0.15 ml then d must be 0.3 ml.

The responses to a, b, c and d are designated A B C and D respectively. It is desirable for the responses of C and D to be slightly more than their standard counterparts A and B to avoid negative signs in the mathematical calculations. The concentration of unknown can be determined graphically (Figure 15) or mathematically using the following formula:

$$\frac{a}{c} \times \text{antilog} \left(\frac{D-B+C-A}{B-A+D-C} \right) \times \log\frac{b}{a}$$

This provides a ratio of potencies of standard to unknown, and from the original concentration of standard the concentration of unknown can therefore be determined.

Agonist potency, affinity constants and efficacy

Activities of different drugs can be expressed as ratios of molar concentration which produce the same response. Commonly a relative potency ratio is expressed to a single drug which is chosen as a standard with which to compare other drugs. Sometimes such comparisons can be misleading especially if the slopes of the log-dose response curves are not the same. In addition the two drugs may have different time courses of action which may be relevant if a predetermined time for measurement of response is used. If either of these factors occur comparisons of relative activities at a single point are meaningless.

Where different drug responses show parallelism and time course is unimportant, measures of relative potency are often made for the response which produces 50% of the maximal response. The terms ED_{50} or EC_{50} (effective dose or concentration producing 50% response) are often used. Where the drug effect is to produce an inhibition of an electrically induced response (e.g. mouse vas deferens, Expt. 5.2) the terms ID_{50} or IC_{50} (inhibitory dose or concentration) are used. In these instances ID_{50} may mean the dose producing 50% inhibition or 50% of maximal inhibition, and this should be stated. For some drugs, maximal inhibition may only be 60% and an ID_{30} (dose producing 30% inhibition) is an alternative when results are not expressed as a % of maximum. An alternative way of expressing ED_{50} is as a

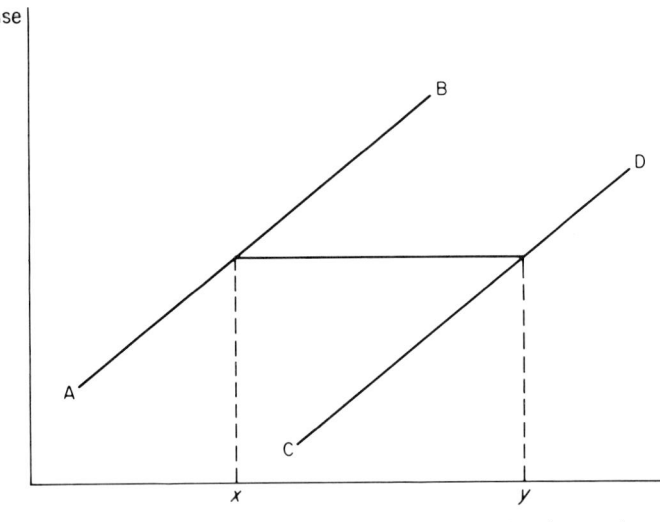

Fig. 15. Graphical determination of unknown concentration for a four point assay. From the graph:

x ml of standard $= y$ ml of unknown taking into account the dilution of standard and unknown to produce the response A, B and C, D respectively.

pD_2 value (i.e. $-$ve $\log_{10}$ of molar concentration of an agonist producing a 50% of maximum response), and this is determined in Expt. 3.3.

Measures of agonist potency of drugs can also be used to determine if agonists are mediating their effects in different preparations through the same receptor using the principle of parallel bioassay. This method is described in greater detail in Expt. 9.4.

The affinity (association) constant of an agonist for its receptor (K_a) can be related to the drug concentration (A) and the proportion of receptors occupied by the drug (y)

$$AK_a = \frac{y}{1-y} \text{ or } y = \frac{AK_a}{1+AK_a}$$

Some workers have used the measures of EC_{50} or pD_2 as determinants of the affinity of an agonist for its receptors. However, this involves the assumption that receptor occupancy is related to the size of biological response measured. Although each *in vitro* system must be considered separately, it is clear that with some of them the size of response is not directly proportional to y. In many systems, there are limitations to the mechanical response of the tissue determined by the method of recording. In addition, bioavailability has to be considered even in the *in vitro* system. Such effects as enzymic breakdown or uptake processes may markedly alter the biological response measured. The concept that biological response is a function not only of receptor occupancy (affinity) but also of the ability of the drug to activate the receptors (efficacy) has generally been upheld and therefore comparing relative activity of agonists in eliciting biological response does not necessarily indicate if one drug binds to a receptor better than another. The stimulus (s) to producing a response has been defined as the product of affinity and efficacy (e), and can be defined as ey. With many full agonist drugs the maximum response of the tissue is produced when the proportion of the receptors occupied is very small. In these circumstances $AK_a = y$ and the stimulus $= eK_a A$.

It may be possible to measure the affinity of an agonist by using an irreversible blocking agent to reduce the proportion of receptors available to the agonist and this method is employed in Expt. 3.5. On the grounds of chemical reactivity certain compounds (e.g. alkylating agents) are thought to combine irreversibly with receptors. In addition, it is assumed that the function of the remaining fraction of receptors is unaffected. If such an agent is employed in sufficient concentration the maximum response of the tissue to an agonist will not be attainable. This reduces the number of bound receptors, and the fraction of receptors remaining is designated q. If the same response is produced by occupation of the same number of receptors before and after the irreversible antagonist then for the agonist receptor interaction before blockade:

$$y = \frac{AK_a}{1 + AK_a}$$

and for the agonist receptor interaction after blockade of a fraction $(1-q)$ of receptors by an irreversible antagonist:

$$y = \left(\frac{A'K_a}{1 + A'K_a}\right) \cdot q$$

therefore

$$\frac{AK_a}{1 + AK_a} = \left(\frac{A'K_a)}{1 + AK_a}\right) \cdot q$$

rearranged

$$\frac{1}{A} = \frac{1}{q}\left(\frac{1}{A'}\right) + K_a\left(\frac{1-q}{q}\right)$$

This equation expresses the relationship between concentrations of agonist (A and A') producing the same magnitude of effect before and after irreversible blockade. A graph of $(1/A)$ against $(1/A')$ should be a straight line. q can be calculated from the slope which equals $(q/1-q)$ and K_a by substituting this value in the equation for the intercept of the $(1/A)$ axis: $K_a = (1-q)/q$.

The strength of stimulus which gives rise to a response which is half the maximal attainable by the tissue is arbitrarily defined as 1. Therefore the efficacy of a drug (which can vary from zero to a large positive number) can be calculated knowing the fraction of receptors it occupies when producing a 50% maximal effect, i.e. when the stimulous strength (s) is unity

therefore
$$s = 1 = ey$$

and
$$y = \frac{A''K_a}{1 + A''K_a}$$

where $A'' =$ concentration of agonist producing a 50% maximal effect before blockade of receptors.

Potent agonists can be expected to produce a half-maximal effect when occupying only a small fraction of the receptor population. Their efficacies are correspondingly high. Antagonists, on the other hand, produce no effect no matter how many receptors they occupy and have zero efficacy. So called partial agonists have activity somewhere between agonists and antagonists and have intermediate values of e.

Measures of antagonism

The relationship between the affinity of competitive antagonists and the biological response is much simpler than that observed for agonists. The affinity constant of an agonist (concentration A) K_a can be related to the affinity constant of an antagonist (concentration B) K_b by the equation

$$AK_a = \frac{y}{1-y}(1 + BK_b)$$

The percentage reduction in the response produced by an antagonist depends on the slope of the dose-response curve and will therefore vary from one preparation to another. This method is, therefore, an unsatisfactory way of attempting to measure antagonism. However, if agonist concentration is increased in the presence of a known concentration of antagonist until the biological response is restored to its original size, then the proportion of receptors occupied (y) should be the same as when agonist alone was used. The original concentration of agonist (a) and the concentration required (A) in the presence of antagonist can be related to K_b by the equation

$$\frac{A}{a} = 1 + BK_b$$

(A/a) is called the dose-ratio for a particular concentration of antagonist (B) and therefore $DR = 1 + BK_b$.

An alternative measure is that of pA_x, which may be defined as the negative log of the molar concentration of a competitive antagonist which will reduce the response of a tissue to a multiple dose of agonist, to that of a single dose of agonist. When the dose-ratio is 2, $B = (1/K_b)$ so pA_2 is identical to log K_b. pA_2 is the negative logarithm of the equilibrium dissociation constant K_e, and sometimes this parameter is used as a measure of the effectiveness of an antagonist against a given agonist (Extp. 5.3): $K_b = (1/K_e)$.

Most quantitative determinations of antagonistic activity depend upon the determination of the dose-ratio. The accuracy of the method depends upon an accurate estimate of the dose-ratio. Most methods involve assays of agonists similar to those already described in the absence and the presence of an antagonist. Equilibration of a tissue with an antagonist may only take a few minutes but as a general rule 15 minutes equilibration is allowed before repeating agonist doses. The smaller the dose-ratio the greater the chance is of inaccurate determinations of K_b. It is best to use concentrations of antagonist which produce dose-ratios > 10. Arunlakshana and Schild (1959) showed that if log $(DR-1)$ is plotted against $-$ log B (i.e. pA_x) a straight line with a negative slope of n is obtained, where the pA_2 value intersects the x-axis (abscissa) i.e. for pA_2,

$$\log (DR - 1) = \log (2 - 1)$$
$$= \log 1$$
$$= 0$$

thus zero on the y-axis (ordinate) $= pA_2$. This method of plotting the dose shift ratio minus one $(DR-1)$ against the negative log of the antagonist concentration $(-\log B, pA_x)$ is known as a 'Schild plot'. If the antagonism is competitive, the graph is a straight line with a negative slope approximating to unity.

At the pA_2 value

$$\log (DR - 1) = \log K_b - npA_2$$
therefore, $\quad \log (2 - 1) = \log K_b - npA_2$
therefore, $\quad 0 = \log K_b - npA_2$
therefore, $\quad npA_2 = \log K_b$
when $n = 1$, $\quad pA_2 = \log K_b$

At the pA_{10} value

$$\log (10 - 1) = \log K_b - npA_{10}$$

$$\log 9 = \log K_b - npA_{10}$$

therefore, $0.9542 = \log K_b - npA_{10}$

when $n = 1$, $0.9542 = \log K_b - pA_{10}$

but $K_b = pA_2$ when $n = 1$

Therefore, for competitive antagonists, $pA_2 - pA_{10} = 0.95$.

However, it is more accurate to test for competitive antagonism via a Schild plot, over a wide range of antagonist concentrations, than to use the above equation. However, the time taken to carry out complete dose-response curves in the absence and presence of at least four concentrations of antagonist allowing 15 minutes for complete equilibration at each concentration, is often prohibitive. A simpler practical model for determining the pA_2 can be used and is described in Expt. 3.4. This method attempts to reduce the response to a double dose of agonist ($2x$) to that of a single dose of agonist (x), in the presence of an antagonist.

Several doses of antagonist are employed for short contact times and the degree of antagonism is expressed as %$2x$ of x. %$2x$ of x is plotted against $\log_{10}$ concentration of antagonist.

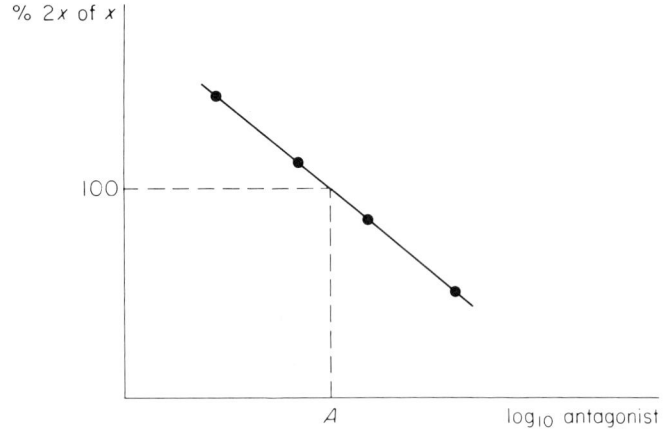

Fig. 16. Graphical Determination of pA_2.

The pA_2 value shown on the graph as A is the point where %$2x$ of x is 100%.

Physiological antagonism and inhibitory assays

In some situations the blocking activity of a drug may be an active process rather than the competitive receptor antagonism already described. In this situation a compound which is by definition an agonist may act antagonistically when compared with a response to another agonist. For example, adrenaline causes relaxation of intestinal muscle by virtue of its activity at adrenergic receptors. Acetylcholine produces contraction of intestine by acting upon muscarinic receptors. Adrenaline is therefore capable of antagonising acetylcholine induced contractions by producing an opposing physiological response. Herein lies the principle of what is termed physiological antagonism. It is not possible to calculate a relationship between the concentrations of acetylcholine and adrenaline for which the response is constant, since the dose-ratio will depend upon the sensitivity of the particular tissue to the two compounds. The log-dose response curves for the two agonists are probably not related to each other. However, the principle of physiological antagonism can be used to determine the concentration of an unknown solution of one of the agonists using an inhibitory assay (Expt. 3.2 and 1.1). Isolated intestinal muscle often has no inherent tone and a direct biological effect of adrenaline is often not observed. However, the relaxation induced by adrenaline can be observed as an inhibition of the contractile response to acetylcholine and an unknown solution of adrenaline can be matched to a standard concentration in terms of the degree of inhibitory activity. Two doses of adrenaline (standard low and standard high) producing inhibitory effects on a submaximal dose of acetylcholine can be compared with two equivalent doses of unknown using the 2×2 assay principle.

Experimental parameters and drugs

See pp. 43 and 44.

Expt. 3.1 Comparison of a bracket assay and a four point assay for the determination of an unknown concentration of histamine using guinea-pig ileum

Set up the ileum as described in Expt. 2.1.

Experimental protocol

1 Determine doses of histamine which produce responses between 25% and 75% of maximum.
2 Determine a dose of unknown which produces a response mid-way between 25% and 75% of maximum.

3 Bracket the unknown dose between two standard doses of histamine producing responses smaller and larger than that produced by the unknown. Attempt to keep the limits of the bracket as close as possible.

4 Choose two doses of histamine standard and two doses of unknown which produce responses between 25% and 75% of maximum ensuring that the dose volume ratio for standards and for unknowns is the same. Designate the four doses A, B, C and D. Show four responses to A, B, C and D using a latin square (p. 56) for randomising the order of dosing.

5 Further accuracy can be achieved by increasing the number of estimates of A, B, C and D using further latin squares.

Estimate the concentration of unknown by 1, graphically using the bracket assay method (p. 55); 2, graphically using the estimate of the mean for the four point assay (p. 56); and 3, using the mathematical formula for four point assay (p. 57).

Expt. 3.2 Determination of an unknown concentration of adrenaline using guinea-pig ileum and an inhibitory assay

Set up the ileum as described in Expt. 2.1.

Experimental protocol

1 Determine a dose of acetylcholine which produces a submaximal response large enough to show measurable inhibition by antagonists and ensure this response is consistent.

2 Add adrenaline and leave in contact with the tissue for 1 minute. Without washing repeat the dose of acetylcholine.

3 Repeat acetylcholine until the response returns to the control level.

4 Repeat 2 using a concentration of adrenaline which will provide a greater or lesser inhibitory effect. An attempt should be made to determine concentrations of adrenaline which produce approximately 30% and 70% inhibition.

5 Repeat 3.

6 Repeat 2-5 for the unknown solution of adrenaline attempting to match as closely as possible the inhibitory effects to those observed with the standards. It is important to keep dose volume ratios for unknown and standard equal (see p. 57).

Calculate the unknown concentration of adrenaline using a graphical method and by the mathematical formula derived for a 2×2 assay (p. 57).

Expt. 3.3 Determination of pD_2 values for acetylcholine, histamine and nicotine on guinea-pig ileum

Set up the ileum as described in Expt. 2.1.

Experimental protocol

1 Carry out full dose-response curves for acetylcholine, histamine and nicotine ensuring that a maximal response is attained for each drug.

Calculate pD_2 values ($-\log_{10}$ of molar concentration of agonist producing a 50% of maximal response) by plotting log dose-response curves for each drug.

Expt. 3.4 Determination of pA_2 for diphenhydramine versus histamine using guinea-pig ileum

Set up the ileum as described in Expt. 2.1. pA_2 values are determined using the method of Lockett and Bartlett (1956).

Experimental protocol

1 Obtain dose related responses to histamine and choose a dose (designated $2x$) which produces a response approximately 70% of maximum.
2 Repeat $2x$ three times to ensure the response is constant followed by three doses of half this concentration (x).
3 Add a dose of diphenhydramine to the bath (choose a dose approximately ten times less than the lowest dose of histamine that produces a measurable response), and leave the antagonist in contact with the preparation for exactly two minutes. Without washing repeat $2x$.
4 Repeat $2x$ until the original response in the absence of antagonist is restored, and three constant responses are obtained.
5 Repeat 3 for at least three doses of antagonist. Choose appropriate concentrations which reduce the response of $2x$ below and above the response observed for x, as well as one point which as closely as possible reduces the response to $2x$ to that of x. Between each dose of antagonist repeat 4.

Calculate the pA_2 value for diphenhydramine versus histamine using the graphical method described on p. 62. The pA_2 value under these experimental conditions will be dependent on the contact time and this must always be stated. Sometimes the sensitivity of the ileum to histamine may change during the course of the experiment. With histamine an increased response for the same dose is often observed during the course of the experiment. A correction factor for such changes should be employed. It must be assumed that any variation of response to $2x$ is linear with respect to the presumed variation of response to x. It is often as well to repeat x at intervals throughout the experiment to ensure this is so. $\% 2x$ of x is calculated for three responses to $2x$ prior to each dose of diphenhydramine. A mean of these three is taken for each set, and the subsequent inhibited response in the presence of antagonist is corrected with respect to the mean of the three reference doses of $2x$ (see 2).

Therefore:

$$\text{corrected } \% \, 2x \text{ of } x = \frac{2x_A}{(\bar{x}_0)} \times \frac{(\overline{2x_0})}{(2x_I)} \times 100\%$$

Where x_0 = mean of original responses to x
   $\overline{2x_0}$ = mean of original responses to $2x$
   $\overline{2x_1}$ = mean of subsequent responses to $2x$
   $2x_A$ = response to $2x$ in presence of antagonist observed after responses to $(2x_1)$.

The pA_2 value must be expressed in molar concentration, and therefore the molecular weight of the diphenhydramine salt must be known if the experiment was carried out using w/v concentrations.

Histamine is a particularly good agonist to choose for these experiments as dose cycles as short as 90 seconds can often be employed without observing tachyphylaxis. Mepyramine is an alternative antagonist but is adsorbed onto glassware. Acetylcholine versus atropine also gives good results.

Expt. 3.5 Determination of the affinity constant and efficacy for histamine and its receptors in isolated guinea-pig ileum using an irreversible antagonist

Set up the ileum as described in Expt. 2.1.

Experimental protocol

1   Carry out a full dose-response curve to histamine with at least three points falling on the linear region of the log dose-response curve. Select a test dose of histamine producing a large, reproducible submaximal contraction.

2 Add phenoxybenzamine to the bath and leave in contact with the tissue for 30 seconds. Repeat the test dose of histamine and after recording the response wash out both drugs thoroughly.

3 Repeat 1.

4 Repeat 2 and 3 several times until a depression of the maximal response is observed.

5 By adjusting the dose of antagonist and/or the duration of exposure obtain two histamine dose response curves: one with a maximum approximately 90% of the original maximal effect and the other approximately 70% of the original.

Calculation of affinity constant

The affinity constant K_a for histamine is calculated thus (see also pp. 57–60).

Plot histamine response versus dose for the curves whose maxima are 90% and 70% of the original maximum. Use these curves to obtain paired values of A and A' (concentration of agonist before and after irreversible blockade) as shown below.

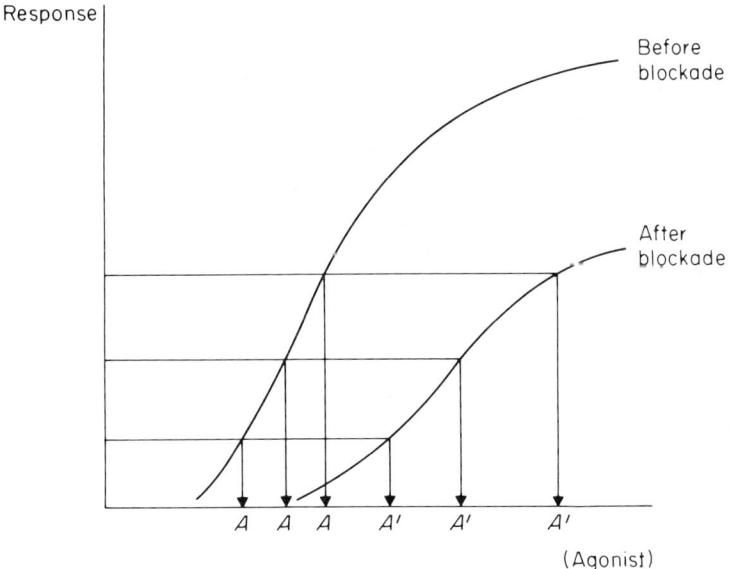

Fig. 17. Graphical determination of A and A' for calculation of affinity constant.

Plot a graph of $(1/A)$ on the ordinate and $(1/A')$ on the abscissa. The slope of this line is equal to

$$q = \frac{\text{concentration of unblocked receptors in the 70\% curve}}{\text{concentration of unblocked receptors in the 90\% curve}}$$

The intercept on the $(1/A)$ axis is used to obtain the value of K_a, where

$$\text{intercept} = K_a \frac{(1-q)}{q}$$

Before calculating K_a convert the units of measurement of the intercept to $(\text{molar})^{-1}$.

Calculation of efficacy

Plot the first histamine log dose-response curve before exposure to phenoxy-benzamine and determine the molar concentration producing a 50% maximal effect (A''). Efficacy e can be calculated from the equation

$$e = \frac{1 + A'' K_a}{A'' K_a}$$

(see p. 60).

Isolated Skeletal Muscle

Introduction

Skeletal muscle is so named because of its anatomical attachment to the skeleton. Other classifications have depended on histological appearance and as skeletal muscle shows cross-striations it is described as striated. However, cardiac muscle is also striated and termed accordingly. It has also been common to describe skeletal muscle as voluntary as there is conscious control of several skeletal muscle movements. Again this terminology is unsatisfactory as the skeletal muscle of the diaphragm which controls respiratory movements is predominantly under involuntary control similar to the smooth muscle movements of the intestine or contraction of cardiac muscle.

Three types of muscle fibre are present in the mammalian muscle: red, intermediate and white, each originally classified by pigmentation resulting from myoglobin content. The classification is now more complex as several differences between the characteristics of each fibre type have been delineated. The muscles of birds and amphibians contain essentially the same three types of fibre. In general, both red and white fibres are fast-contracting whilst intermediate fibres are slow-contracting. Skeletal muscles are innervated by somatic motor nerves which are fast-conducting and myelineated. The axons of these motoneurones pass without interruption from the central nervous system to the muscles. There is extensive branching and a single axon innervates many muscle fibres. The motoneurone together with the muscle fibre it innervates is called a motor unit and the junctional region where the nerve endings contact the muscle is known as the motor end-plate. Acetylcholine is the neurotransmitter released from all somatic motor nerves and the receptors which mediate its effect are nicotinic (though importantly dissimilar from nicotinic receptors at ganglia).

Most mammalian fibres receive their innervation at a single end plate region. Where this is the case, the innervation is described as focal. In contrast, multiply-innervated fibres, which are common in amphibia and birds, receive a dense innervation and as many as 70–80 end plate regions may be present in each muscle fibre. Multiply-innervated fibres are usually of the slow-contracting type.

69

The frog rectus abdominis (Exp. 4.1–4.4) contains both multiply-innervated and focally-innervated fibres but the characteristics of response are typical of multiply-innervated fibres. The effect of stimulation produces depolarisation of small areas of muscle fibre at the nerve ending and there is no action potential generated. All of the electrical disturbance is localised to the axon terminal and is transmitted inwards by the transverse tubule system of the sarcoplasmic reticulum. The inefficiency of this system probably accounts for the relatively slow rate of contraction of the myofibrils. The slow and maintained contraction which is observed with agonist drugs is called contracture. In order to ensure that the muscle returns to baseline, a stretching weight of 0.5–1 g is applied after drug additions.

As frogs are cold-blooded the rectus preparation is used at room temperature. A specialised frog Ringer solution is also employed, equivalent to 0.6% saline which is iso-osmotic for frog tissue. All drug dilutions should therefore be made in 0.6% saline.

The rat phrenic nerve hemi-diaphragm preparation (Expt. 4.5 and 4.6) is a good example of focally-innervated skeletal muscle. The response to nervous stimulation is fast contraction and a characteristic skeletal muscle twitch is observed. In contrast to the rectus muscle, release of acetylcholine onto the specialised end-plate region causes a local depolarisation termed the end-plate potential. When this depolarisation reaches a threshold level a propagated action potential is set up in the muscle fibre causing it to contract. The contractile response of the fibre is all or none as distinct from the graded contractions observed in the rectus muscle or, for example, smooth muscle preparations.

The phrenic nerve hemidiaphragm preparation allows observation of nerve-mediated muscle contraction and its modification by drugs. It works perfectly well at both 37°C and 20°C though effects on the cholinesterase system are often masked at room temperature. The tissue will survive for several hours if well aerated and either Krebs solution or Tyrode (containing double glucose) are suitable Ringers.

The chick biventer cervicis preparation (Expt. 4.7) contains both slow and fast (twitch) muscle fibres. It is thus ideal to demonstrate drug effects that would be seen in both rat diaphragm and frog rectus. In response to stimulation of nerves which lie in the tendon supplying the muscle it gives twitch responses but will also produce a contracture to agonist drugs.

Drugs

Cholinergic agonists

Drugs which stimulate nicotinic receptors such as acetylcholine cause contracture of slow muscle fibres and have no effect, or facilitate twitch responses of fast fibres. At high concentrations or in the presence of anticholinesterase drugs the twitch response is inhibited due to deplorisation block (see below).

Neuromuscular blockers

Two types of neuromuscular blocking drugs (competitive or non-depolarising and depolarising) can be studied using isolated skeletal muscle preparations. In fast-conducting, focally-innervated preparations competitive neuromuscular blockers such as tubocurarine, block the twitch response. The antagonism is competitive and can be reversed by increasing the acetylcholine concentration at the synapse using an anticholinesterase drug such as neostigmine or physostigmine. In contrast, blockers of the depolarising type such as suxamethonium or decamethonium cause neuromuscular block, which is sometimes preceded by transient fasciculation, and is unaffected or worsened by anticholinesterase drugs. These neuromuscular blocking drugs produce a persistent depolarisation, and their effects are long-lasting.

In slow-contracting, multiply-innervated fibres response to drugs such as acetylcholine can be blocked by competitive neuromuscular blockers. In contrast to fast fibres there is no such thing as depolarisation block. Suxamethonium and decamethonium themselves produce contracture and have no blocking activity on acetylcholine induced responses.

Anticholinesterases

Anticholinesterases potentiate acetylcholine responses in slow contracting multiply-innervated muscles. This facilitation in fast fibres can lead to depolarisation block. Only competitive neuromuscular blockade can be reversed by anticholinesterase drugs.

Sympathomimetics

Sympathomimetic amines in high doses can produce skeletal muscle tremor. Depending on the species and the experimental conditions sympathomimetics can be shown to influence the muscle fibres themselves, the muscle spindles, the neuromuscular transmitting process and conduction in the nerve. Their effects differ to some extent according to whether the muscle is fatigued or non-fatigued. In mammalian fast fibres a facilitation of twitch-response can be observed with adrenaline, isoprenaline or salbutamol. It is generally agreed that this effect is mediated via β_2-receptors and is sensitive to antagonism with β-blocking drugs such as propanolol. In frog rectus muscle sympathomimetics are normally ineffective.

Experimental parameters

Organ bath	Frog rectus abdominis	10 ml
	Chick biventer cervicis	20 ml
	Rat phrenic nerve diaphragm	100 ml
Ringer solution	Frog	Frog Ringer
	Rat	Tyrode (double glucose) or Krebs
	Chick	Krebs
Aeration	Frog	Air
	Rat and Chick	95% O_2/5% CO_2
Bath temperature	Frog	20°C
	Rat	20°C or 37°C
	Chick	37°C
Recording	Frog	Isotonic
	Rat and Chick	Isometric
Resting tension	Frog	0.5 g (+1 g stretching wt)
	Rat	0.5 g
	Chick	0.3 g
Equilibration period	Frog	30–45 minutes
	Rat and Chick	15–30 minutes
Dose cycle	Frog	4–7 minutes
	Rat and Chick	10 minutes
Contact time	Frog	1–1½ minutes
	Rat and Chick	3–6 minutes
Stimulus parameters	Rat	Pulse width 0.5 ms Voltage < 15 V Frequency 0.1 Hz
	Chick	Pulse width 1–2 ms Voltage < 15 V Frequency 0.1 Hz

Drugs (final bath concentration: starting dose)

	Frog	Rat	Chick
Acetylcholine	250 ng/ml	100 μg/ml	5 μg/ml
Adrenaline			5 μg/ml
Carbachol	1 μg/ml		
Methacholine	5 μg/ml		
Neostigmine		1 μg/ml	50 ng/ml
Physostigmine	10 μg/ml		
Suxamethonium	250 ng/ml	2 μg/ml	100 ng/ml
(+)-Tubocurarine	1 μg/ml	1 μg/ml	10 μg/ml

Expt. 4.1 Cholinomimetic drugs and the frog rectus abdominis muscle

Decapitate a frog after stunning and pith the animal using a pithing needle. This procedure simply involves inserting the needle into the spinal cord. Rotate the needle until the base of the cord is reached and ensure that leg reflexes are absent. Place the frog, ventral side up, on a cork board and make a cut in mid ventral line of the trunk. Separate the skin along this mid line, expose the recti muscles which lie underneath and moisten the tissues with Frog Ringer. Make two longitudinal cuts on either side of the xiphoid cartilage and follow the line of the recti muscles to their attachment to the pubis. The striated appearance of the recti muscles makes it easy to distinguish them from the surrounding pectoralis posterior muscles at the upper end and the obliques externis muscle at the lower end. Make a transverse cut through the xiphoid cartilage and whilst supporting the muscles by forceps, free the tissue from its attachment to the pubis. Transfer the recti muscles to a petri dish containing Frog Ringer and separate them from the xiphoid cartilage. The two muscles can be set up together but it is best to separate them by making a longitudinal cut along the linea alba. Two rectus preparations can therefore be obtained from one frog. Pass threads through the muscle at both top and bottom and attach the bottom thread to the tissue holder. Transfer the mounted preparation to the organ bath and attach the top thread to an isotonic transducer. In addition to the resting tension applied to this tissue it is necessary to apply a further stretching weight to ensure the muscle returns to its baseline after drug-induced contracture. For isotonic transducers employing a lever system pivoted on a fulcrum hang a 1 g weight from a thread on the opposite side to the attachment of the tissue, equidistant from the

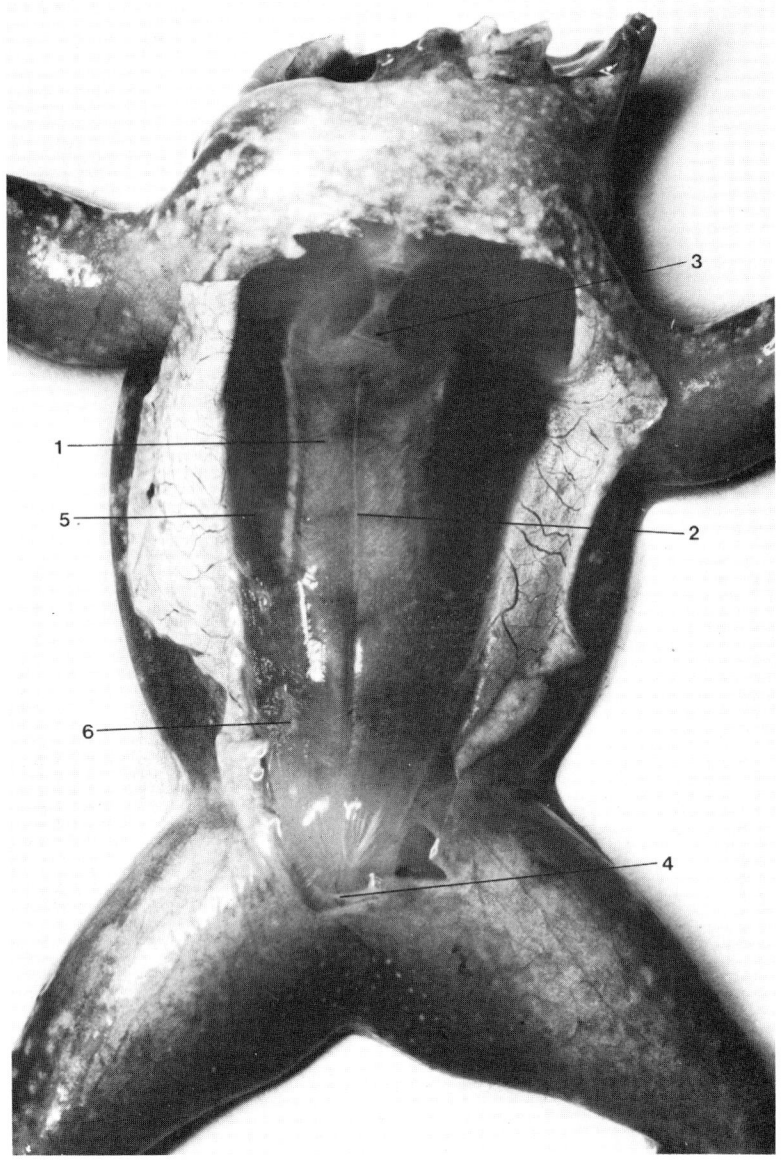

Fig. 18. Dissection of the frog rectus abdominis muscles.

The skin is cut exposing the rectus abdominis muscles (1) separated by the linea alba (2). The muscles are dissected from the xiphoid cartilage (3) to the pubis (4) leaving the surrounding pectoralis posterior muscle (5) and the obliquis externis muscle (6).

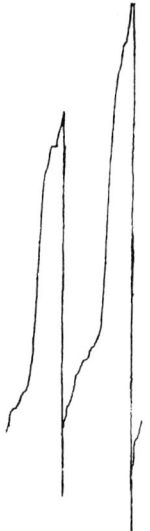

Fig. 19. Responses of the frog rectus abdominis muscle to acetylcholine (▲ 500 ng/ml, △ 1 μg/ml).

fulcrum. Leave this weight hanging to stretch the muscle at all times, except when running a baseline trace and observing a drug response. At these times locate the weight (still attached to its thread) on a suitable part of the apparatus where it will not interfere with the lever movement of the transducer. Some isotonic transducers use spring arrangements hung from the cantilever of a strain gauge. When these are used, calibrate the transducer and chart trace as you would for isometric measurement (p. 7) marking two points on the chart recorder trace, one equivalent to the resting tension and the other equivalent to the resting tension plus 1 g. Adjust the transducer with the tissue attached so that the chart recorder pen corresponds to the 1.5 g calibration point.

Before each drug addition ensure that the baseline is relatively flat since removal of the stretching weight will initially produce an increase in muscle tone.

Experimental protocol

1 Show dose related responses to acetylcholine and construct a full dose response curve.

2 Repeat 1 for carbachol.

3 Repeat 1 for methacholine.

This experiment should show the lack of activity of muscarinic agonists such as methacholine on neuromuscular preparations. Carbachol is less potent than acetylcholine on this tissue but the responses are often more prolonged. This may be related to the resistance to breakdown by cholinesterase enzymes.

Expt. 4.2 Competitive and depolarising neuromuscular blocking drugs and the frog rectus abdominis muscle

Set up the rectus muscle as described in Expt. 4.1.

Experimental protocol

1 Show dose related responses to acetylcholine and choose a test dose which produces a large submaximal response.
2 Repeat 1 for suxamethonium.
3 Repeat the test dose of acetylcholine.
4 Add (+)-tubocurarine to the organ bath and leave in contact with the tissue for 1 minute and without washing repeat 3.
5 Repeat the acetylcholine test dose until the responses returns to the control level.
6 Repeat 3, 4 and 5 for the test dose of suxamethonium.
7 Repeat the test dose of acetylcholine.
8 Add physostigmine and leave in contact with the tissue for 1 minute, immediately followed without washing by (+)-tubocurarine for a further period of 1 minute. In the presence of both physostigmine and (+)-tubocurarine repeat 7.
9 Repeat 5.
10 Repeat 7, 8 and 9 for the test dose of suxamethonium.

This experiment should show that responses to cholinergic agonists such as acetylcholine are antagonised by competitive neuromuscular blocking drugs such as (+)-tubocararine and that this blockade can be reversed by anticholinesterase compounds such as physostigmine which inhibit the breakdown of acetylcholine. In contrast suxamethonium which exhibits depolarising neuromuscular blockade produces only contracture in slow muscle fibre preparations. Like acetylcholine, the contracture is antagonised by (+)-tubocurarine but not reversed by physostigmine since suxamethonium is not a substrate for acetylcholinesterase.

Expt. 4.3 Effect of cholinesterase enzymes on acetylcholine and carbachol activity using the frog rectus abdominis muscle as an assay preparation

Set up the rectus muscle as described in Expt. 4.1. Dilute whole blood and plasma 1:10 with Frog Ringer. The source of either is not important but expired human blood is useful when large quantities are required. Plasma can be prepared by centrifugation of whole blood at 2000–3000 g for 15 minutes. Set up tubes for incubation in accordance with the following table but do not add the whole blood or plasma until you are ready to start your timed incubations.

Tube no	Acetylcholine 1 mg/ml	Carbachol 1 mg/ml	Frog Ringer	Whole blood 1:10*	Plasma 1:10*	Physo-stigmine 3 μg/ml
1	1 ml	—	2 ml	—	—	—
2	1 ml	—	1 ml	1 ml	—	—
3	1 ml	—	1 ml	—	1 ml	—
4	1 ml	—	—	1 ml	—	1 ml
5	1 ml	—	—	—	1 ml	1 ml
6	—	1 ml	2 ml	—	—	—
7	—	1 ml	1 ml	1 ml	—	—
8	—	1 ml	1 ml	—	1 ml	—
9	—	1 ml	—	1 ml	—	1 ml
10	—	1 ml	—	—	1 ml	1 ml

* Add last to begin incubations

Experimental protocol

1 Determine a concentration of acetylcholine and carbachol that produces a large submaximal response.

2 Ensure that diluted whole blood or plasma have no effect on the preparation by adding volumes equivalent to those which will be added from incubation samples.

3 Begin incubations at 37°C, in the order shown in the table, on a staggered time cycle so that aliquots may be removed and assayed at 0, 10 and 30 minutes from each tube. Choose a volume for assay which will be equivalent to the concentration determined in 1.

The experiment should show that responses to acetylcholine are reduced or even abolished in a time-dependent manner by incubation with whole blood (which contains acetylcholinesterase) or plasma (which contains plasmacholinesterase). Since physostigmine inhibits the activity of both cholinesterase enzymes the loss of activity does not occur when this drug is included in the incubation sample. In addition, physostigmine blocks cholinesterase enzymes present in the rectus muscle itself and may therefore even potentiate the response to acetylcholine. Carbachol in contrast is resistant to enzymic breakdown by both acetylcholinesterase and plasmacholinesterase and its activity should remain unaltered.

The sensitivity of the rectus muscle to cholinomimetics can vary quite considerably but usually aliquot volumes will fall between 0.05 ml and 1 ml if the 1 mg/ml stock concentration is used for incubations.

Expt. 4.4 Hydrolysis of suxamethonium by plasma cholinesterase using the frog rectus abdominis muscle as an assay preparation

Set up the rectus muscle as described in Expt. 4.1 and prepare plasma as described in Expt. 4.3. Prepare incubation tubes for suxamethonium (1 mg/ml) in accordance with the following table but do not add plasma until you are ready to start your timed incubations.

Tube no	Suxamethonium 1 mg/ml	Frog Ringer	Plasma	Physostigmine 3 µg/ml
1	1 ml	2 ml	—	—
2	1 ml	1 ml	1 ml	—
3	1 ml	—	1 ml	1 ml

Experimental protocol

1   Determine a concentration of suxamethonium that produces a large submaximal response.

2   Ensure that the plasma has no effect on the preparation by adding volumes equivalent to those which will be added from incubation samples.

3   Begin incubations at 37°C, in the order shown in the table, on a staggered time cycle so that aliquots may be removed from each tube and assayed at 0, 10 and 30 minutes. Choose a volume for assay which will be equivalent to the concentration determined in 1.

Suxamethonium is hydrolysed by plasma cholinesterase and although this hydrolysis is much slower than that of acetylcholine it is an important determinant in terminating the action of this drug. This experiment should show the loss of activity of suxamethonium, in a time-dependent manner when incubated with plasma. Physostigmine which inhibits both plasma and acetylcholinesterase should prevent the hydrolysis.

Expt. 4.5 Neuromuscular blocking drugs and the rat phrenic nerve hemidiaphragm preparation

The preparation is based on the method of Bulbring (1946). Kill a rat by stunning followed by exsanguination. Lay the animal on its back and remove the fur and skin covering the upper part of the abdomen and thorax. Remove the muscle layers covering the chest and expose the rib cage. Lift the rib cage along the midline with a pair of forceps and make an incision half way between the xiphisternum and the neck. Examine inside the thoracic cavity to ensure that the phrenic nerves are not adhering to the chest-wall as this occasionally happens. If this is the case, gently dislodge the nerves. Make lateral cuts on either side of the midline incision, parallel to the ribs, and fill the cavity with Ringer solution. Lift the caudal edge of the incised rib cage and remove all the ribs except the one attached to the diaphragm on the animal's left side. The left phrenic nerve is always chosen first as it is easier to dissect. The right phrenic nerve lies alongside the inferior vena cava. Remove the upper part of the rib cage up to the neck to facilitate dissection of the nerve. Remove the xiphisternum and make an incision from this central point

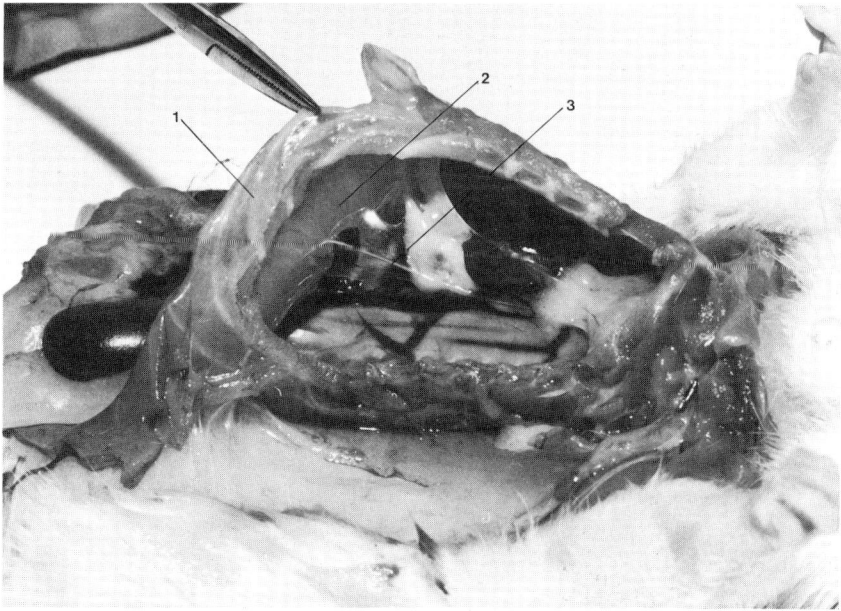

Fig. 20. Dissection of left rat hemidiaphragm and phrenic nerve.
The rib cage is cut away leaving a single rib (1) for attachment of the diaphragm (2) to the tissue holder. The phrenic nerve (3) is dissected out.

vertically to where the diaphragm attaches to the body wall. Cut the hemidiaphragm laterally from its attachment to the body wall so freeing the preparation from the animal. Take care to avoid the phrenic nerve and ensure that the nerve is not stretched. Hold the diaphragm preparation by the remaining rib and dissect the phrenic nerve as far back as possible. A length of 3–4 cm is usually sufficient. Place the nerve and muscle in a petri dish containing Ringer solution and trim any large amounts of connective tissue from the nerve. Do not be over zealous with this procedure; the nerve will function perfectly well with some connective tissue covering it and it is very easy to damage the nerve with forceps and scissors. Tie a piece of cotton to the tip of the tendonous tissue at the apex of the diaphragm preparation for attachment to the transducer. Attach another cotton to the top of the phrenic nerve to facilitate the location of the nerve over the electrode. It is best to attach the preparation to a combined specialised tissue holder and electrode which are available commercially. Locate the rib on the tissue holder and secure the preparation with the mounting bar. Gently pull the nerve across the sliding jaw-hook electrode and close the jaw to secure the nerve. Transfer the mounted preparation to an organ bath, secure the holder and electrode, and attach the muscle to the transducer. Ensure that the preparation is well aerated. Commence stimulation immediately and maintain throughout the experiment, except during washing.

Experimental protocol

1   Show the neuromuscular blocking effects of a single dose of (+)-tubocurarine and suxamethonium. Leave in contact with the tissue for 5 minutes, wash the preparation and wait until the twitch responses return to normal.
2   Repeat 1 except at 3 minutes add neostigmine.
3   Show the effect of a single dose of acetylcholine.
4   Repeat 3 except at 3 minutes add neostigmine.

The experiment should show the neuromuscular blocking activity of (+)-tubocurarine and suxamethonium. Suxamethonium block may be preceded by a transient facilitation of the twitch, and the block is unaffected or worsened by anticholinesterase drugs. In contrast (+)-tubocurarine block should be readily reversed by neostigmine. It may be possible to observe depolarisation block with large amounts of acetylcholine especially in the presence of an anticholinesterase.

The onset and offset of drug responses is very slow and it is not recommended that dose response curves are carried out. The effect of anticholinesterase drugs is sometimes masked when the experiment is performed at room

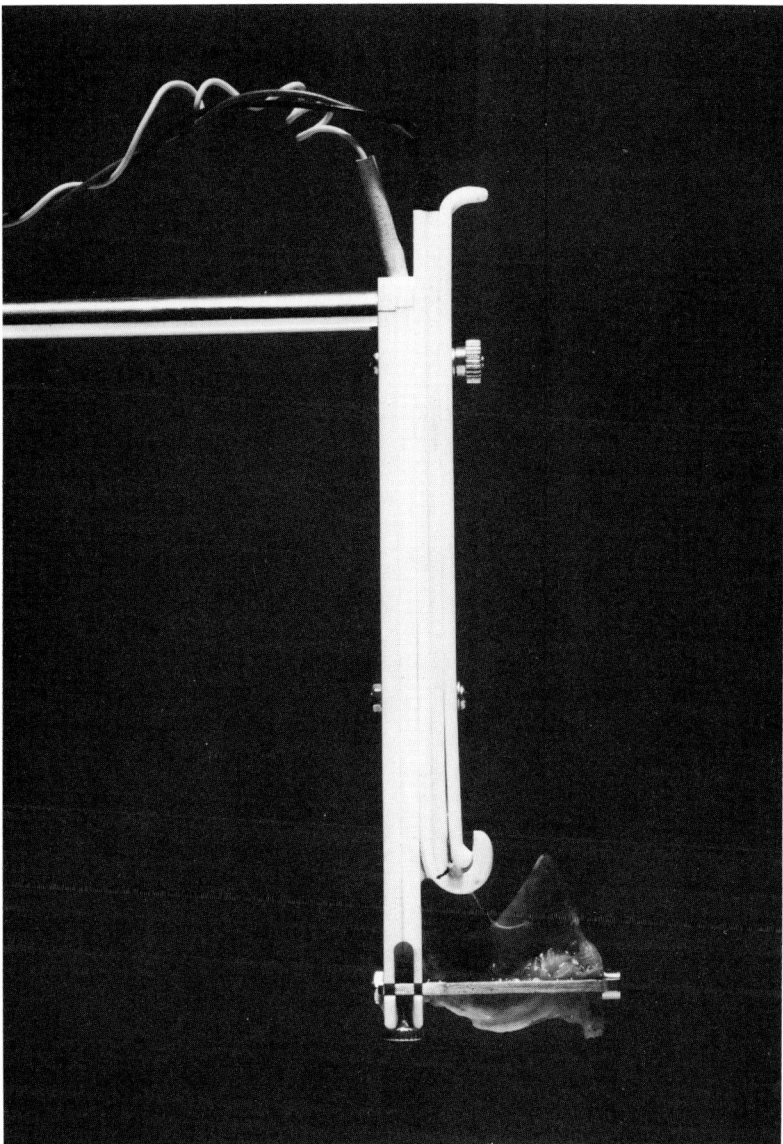

Fig. 21. Mounted diaphragm-phrenic nerve preparation.
The rib is secured in the mounting bar of the tissue holder and the nerve passed over the integral jaw electrode.

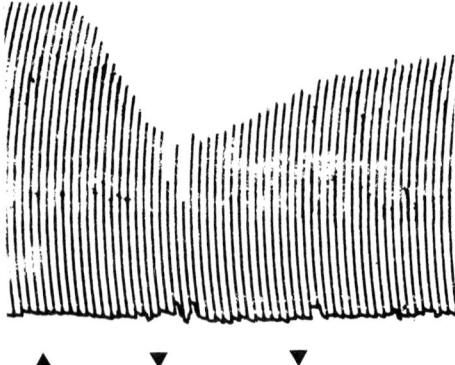

Fig. 22. Response of the stimulated phrenic nerve – rat hemidiaphragm preparation to tubocurarine (▲ 4 μg/ml, 0.1 Hz ▼ Wash).

temperature. If time permits it is an interesting exercise to study drug effects at 20°C and 37°C on this preparation.

Expt. 4.6 The effect of neuromuscular blocking drugs on tetanic responses of the rat phrenic nerve hemidiaphragm preparation

Set up the muscle as described in Expt. 4.5.

Experimental protocol

1 Stimulate the nerve at 0.1 Hz until constant responses are obtained. Increase the stimulus frequency to 40 Hz for 30 seconds and then return to a rate of 0.1 Hz.
2 Add (+)-tubocurarine. When an approximately 70% inhibition of the twitch has occurred increase the stimulus frequency to 40 Hz for 30 seconds and then return to 0.1 Hz. Wash the preparation after a further one minute.
3 When 0.1 Hz twitches have returned to their control level repeat 2 for suxamethonium.

Tetanic responses are observed at a frequency of 40 Hz and it may be possible to observe post-tetanic potentiation of the 0.1 Hz response. This effect is probably due to increased acetylcholine release which occurs in response to single nerve impulses and therefore increases the number of muscle fibres contracting. The tension of tetanic responses observed during competitive neuromuscular blockade rapidly wanes. Tetanus is therefore usually depressed and unsustained. After tetanus single twitches should be temporarily increased in tension due to increased acetylcholine release. In contrast during depolarisation block the tension of tetanus, though depressed, remains sustained. After tetanus, the single twitches are neither increased nor further depressed. The increased acetylcholine released post-tetanically sustains depolarisation block. These effects should be demonstrated in this experiment.

Expt. 4.7 Neuromuscular blocking drugs and the innervated biventer cervicis preparation of the chick

The preparation is set up based on the method of Ginsborg and Warriner (1960). Anaesthetise a chick with sodium pentobarbitone 6 mg/100 g intramuscularly. When the corneal reflex is abolished, pluck the back of the neck and make an incision in the skin along the midline, from the skull to below the base of the neck. Placing the neck over a cotton reel or a tube of similar dimensions aids dissection. Identify the two biventer cervicis muscles which lie on either side of the midline and moisten the tissues with some Ringer solution. Be careful to select the correct tissues, the biventer cervicis are flanked on the outside by thicker semispinalis muscles. Carefully free the upper part of the muscle from surrounding tissue and tie a thread at the uppermost part of the tendon which attaches to the muscle. Apply minimum tension using this thread, and dissect out the caudal belly of the muscle to where the lower tendon attaches to the supraspinous ligament. Both upper and lower tendonous regions are easily identifiable by their silvery white colour. Transfer the preparation to a petri dish containing Ringer solution and tie a thread around the lower tendon. Attach this thread to a tissue holder and transfer the preparation to an organ bath. Gently pull the upper thread through a ring electrode (biventer cervicis electrodes are commercially available) and secure the electrode in position around the upper tendon where the nerve supplying the muscle is located. Attach the upper thread to the transducer. It may be necessary to resite the electrode to obtain the best twitch response once the muscle is under resting tension.

Experimental protocol

1 Simulate at a frequency of 0.1 Hz using supramaximal stimuli. Add adrenaline and observe the response.

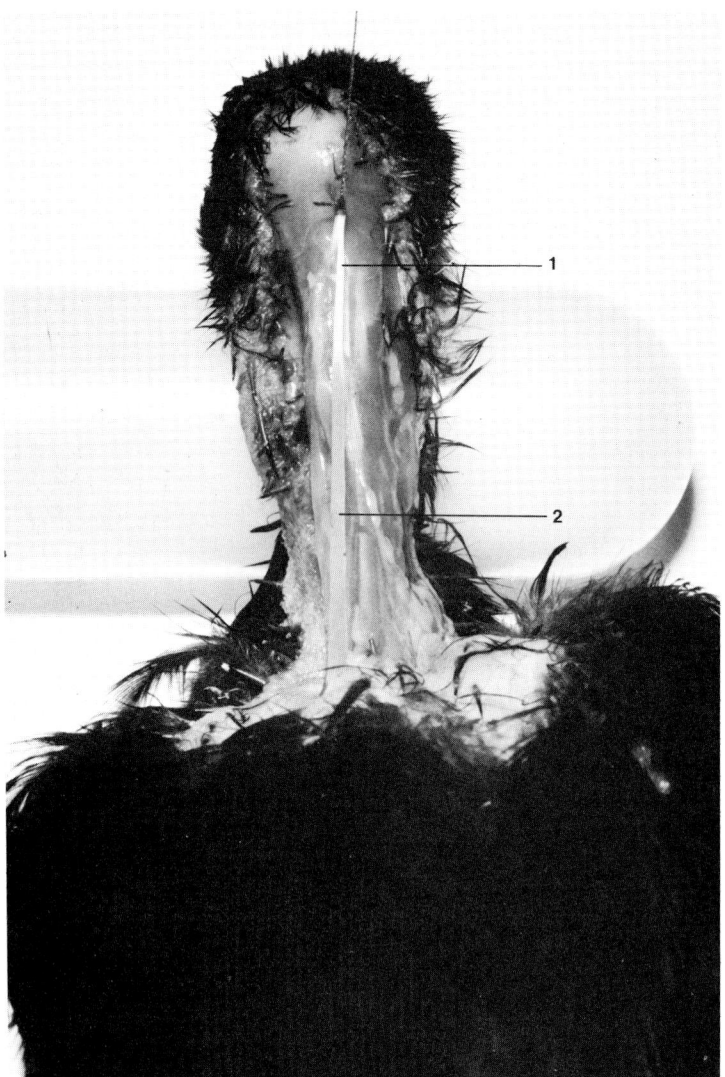

Fig. 23. Dissection of the chick biventer cervicis.
A tie is placed around the tendon (1) and tension applied to the biventer cervicis muscle (2) to aid dissection.

2 Repeat 1 using submaximal stimuli obtained by reducing the stimulator voltage.

3 Using supramaximal stimuli show dose related effects of acetylcholine.

4 Add neostigmine at a dose that does not induce contracture (5 ng–50 ng/ml) and repeat a dose of acetylcholine that produced a submaximal response.

5 Show the neuromuscular blocking effect of a single dose of suxamethonium.

6 Repeat 5 for (+)-tubocurarine.

7 Repeat 6, and before full neuromuscular blockade is observed add neostigmine.

8 Repeat (7) for suxamethonium.

The experiment should show both contracture and depolarisation block for acetylcholine and suxamethonium which is enhanced by neostigmine. In contrast (+)-tubocurarine has no activity on the slow muscle fibres and the neuromuscular blockade of the twitch fibres is reversed by neostigmine.

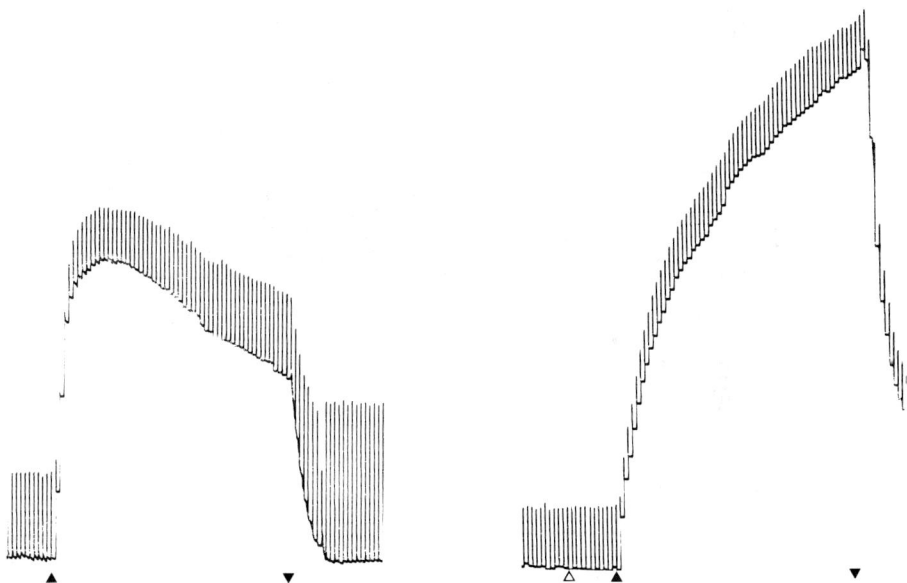

Fig. 24. Responses of the innervated biventer cervicis preparation of the chick to electrical stimulation (0.1 Hz) and to acetylcholine (▲ 4 μg/ml; ▼ wash). Effect of pyridostigmine (△ 80 ng/ml).

Isolated Vas Deferens

Introduction

The use of isolated vas deferens preparations in pharmacological research has grown enormously in the last decade. The guinea-pig vas deferens-hypogastric nerve preparation was first described in the early 1960s and requires no specialised apparatus to carry out the experiment. The more recently described preparations, such as the field stimulated vasa deferentia of the mouse, rat and rabbit require the provision of stimulators with high current outputs, which are more expensive than the simple 'student' stimulator. It is possible to build simple constant current generators relatively cheaply which can be connected to basic stimulators. The stimulator then provides the pulse width and frequency of stimulation whilst the generator determines the output of the pulses. A circuit diagram of a constant current generator is given in Fig. 4 (p. 13).

Autonomic innervation of the vas deferens appears to be exclusively sympathetic. In many species it has a very dense noradrenergic innervation, which is atypical since the ganglion cells lie close to the innervated tissue. These short adrenergic neurones can be demonstrated in the nerve muscle preparation of the guinea-pig (Expt. 5.1). Though the noradrenaline content of the mouse vas deferens is high there is some controversy as to whether noradrenaline is the excitatory motor transmitter. Studies of the transversely bisected vas deferens have suggested the existence of an adrenergic component predominant in the epididymal portion and a non-adrenergic component predominant in the prostatic half. In the whole vas the contractile response to nerve stimulation is resistant to reduction by α-adrenoceptor antagonists at concentrations which increase the nerve induced output of noradrenaline. One suggestion to explain this is that there are a separate set of non-adrenergic nerves of which the transmitter is unknown.

The vas deferens consists of three muscle layers whose relative thickness vary from species to species and from one end to the other. There is a layer of circular muscle which is bounded between an inner and outer longitudinal muscle coat. In all experiments only contractions of the longitudinal muscle fibres are measured, and considerable tension can be generated in this layer.

Since vasa deferentia have narrow lumens, transmural stimulation is not suitable and mouse, rat and rabbit preparations contract well in response to field stimulation. The design of electrodes will have a bearing on the tension generated and also possibly on the sensitivity to drugs (see p. 11). The author's preference is for linear platinum gutter electrodes fixed parallel to the tissue. All field stimulated responses are due to stimulation of intramural nerves and can be blocked by tetrodotoxin. It is very difficult to stimulate the muscle directly using single pulse field stimulation and even at current strengths of 800 mA a pulse width > 10 ms is necessary. Field stimulated responses can be achieved with single, double (twin) or trains of pulses. Double pulses are preferred as the tension generated by the tissue for a given current is substantially greater than that seen with single pulses. Though trains of pulses will generate still further tension, a great deal of criticism has been levelled at this method and it is often considered as unphysiological. The responses of the rat vas to α-adrenoceptor antagonists are dependent on whether single or trains of pulses are used, and the inhibitory actions of opioids on the mouse vas are greatly reduced when employing train stimulation. Tensions generated by the mouse vas deferens in response to field stimulation can be as low as 100–200 mg and high gain preamplifiers with adequate filtering circuits are necessary for recording responses.

Vasa deferentia preparations require careful handling and the use of forceps should be kept to a minimum. At room temperature they survive well without oxygen and there is no rush to get the tissues to an oxygenated bath. The contractile response of both the mouse and rat vas deferens to field stimulation is markedly increased by omitting the magnesium from the Krebs. In addition the responses to opioid drugs are often more constant in magnesium-free Krebs.

The mouse vas deferens preparation can be regarded as the isolated tissue of the pharmacologist's dream. It responds to several drugs and possesses a complement of drug receptors paralleled only by intestinal muscle. A great deal of research effort in identifying pre- and post-synaptic α-adrenoceptors has been centred around the mouse vas. In addition, there has been extensive use of this preparation in studies of multiple opioid receptors.

Drugs

Adrenergic agonists and antagonists

The mouse vas deferens possesses both α_1- and α_2- adrenoceptors at post- and pre-synaptic sites respectively. The characteristics of response to α-adrenoceptor agonists are markedly different and dependent on their selectivity for the pre- and post-synaptic sites. Stimulation of α_2-adrenoceptors by clonidine and low concentrations of noradrenaline inhibit the field stimulated twitch response. At higher concentrations of noradrenaline a contracture is super-imposed on the twitch responses and this post-synaptic response is due to stimulation of α_1-adrenoceptors. Similarly phenylephrine (a selective α_1-adrenoceptor agonist) produces a contracture but, unlike noradrenaline, it potentiates the twitch response. These α-adrenoceptor responses are blocked by selective α_1- and α_2-adrenoceptor antagonists (Expt. 5.4).

Responses to noradrenaline are unaffected by β-adrenoceptor antagonists. However, β_2-adrenoceptors do appear to be present in the mouse vas since isoprenaline and salbutamol inhibit the twitch response, an effect blocked by propranolol but not practolol.

Inhibitory pre-synaptic dopamine receptors probably exist in the rat vas but not in vas deferens of the guinea-pig or mouse. However, dopamine inhibits the twitch response in the mouse vas by virtue of its agonist activity at α-adrenoceptors. Dopamine effects are blocked by yohimbine and phentolamine.

Indirectly-acting sympathomimetics

Tyramine, which releases noradrenaline, produces a contraction of the rat vas deferens which can be blocked by α-adrenocepytor antagonists. In addition, like noradrenaline, tyramine inhibits the field-stimulated response as does the noradrenaline uptake blocker cocaine. The effects of tyramine and cocaine are studied in Expt. 5.8.

Opioids

The mouse vas deferens possesses both μ- and δ-opioid receptors. Stimulation of opioid receptors inhibits the twitch response by pre-synaptic inhibition of noradrenaline release. The relative proportions of these two receptor types vary from strain to strain and these differences are investigated in Expt. 5.6. Many of the opioid alkaloids such as morphine act at μ-opioid receptors whilst the endogenous enkephalin pentapeptides are relatively selective for the δ-opioid receptor which predominates in the mouse vas. Differences in K_e values for the opioid antagonist naloxone, against morphine and the enkephalins, provided early confirmatory evidence for the existence of multiple opioid receptor sites. These differences are shown in Expt. 5.3.

The rat vas deferens also possesses μ- and δ-opioid receptors whilst the rabbit appears to contain almost exclusively k-opioid receptors. The rat vas deferens is particularly well-equipped to degrade the enkephalin pentapeptides and the inhibitory effects of these opioids is markedly increased by peptidase inhibition (Expt. 5.7).

Autacoids

Histamine and some prostaglandins inhibit the twitch responses of the mouse vas deferens. As for opioids the inhibitory effects of histamine are strain dependent. The effect of histamine appears to be mediated via H_2-receptors and is blocked by cimetidine. It is important to note that some H_2-antagonists such as metiamide block pre-synaptic α_2-adrenoceptors in the vas.

Experimental parameters

Organ bath	Guinea-pig	50 ml
	Mouse	3 ml
	Rat	5 ml
Ringer solution	Guinea-pig and Rat	Krebs
	Mouse	Mg^{++}-free Krebs
Aeration		95% O_2/5% CO_2
Bath temperature	Guinea-pig	32°C
	Mouse and Rat	36°C
Recording	Guinea-pig	Isotonic
	Mouse and Rat	Isometric
Resting tension	Guinea-pig	1 g
	Mouse	0.2 g
	Rat	0.5 g
Equilibration period		45 minutes
Dose cycle	Guinea-pig	2–4 minutes
	Mouse	7–10 minutes
	Rat	7–10 minutes
Contact time	Mouse	1–2 minutes
	Rat	1–2 minutes
Stimulus parameters	Guinea-pig	Pulse width 2 ms
		Voltage < 5V
		Frequency 5–30 Hz
		Stimulus Duration 10 s

Stimulus parameters	Mouse	Double pulse
		Pulse width 1 ms
		Pulse spacer 75 ms
		Voltage > 100 V
		(> 100 mA)
		Frequency 0.1 Hz
	Expt. 5.7	Pulse width 1 ms
		Voltage > 100 V
		(> 150 mA)
		Frequency 0.1 Hz
	Expt. 5.8	Pulse width 1 ms
		Voltage > 100 V
		(> 150 mA)
		Frequency 0.02 Hz

Drugs (final bath concentration: starting dose)

	Guinea-pig	Mouse	Rat
ATP		10 μg/ml	
Atropine			1 μg/ml
Cocaine			5 μg/ml
Clonidine		30 ng/ml	
(D-Ala^2, D-Leu^5)-enkephalin			10 ng/ml
Dopamine		200 ng/ml	
Guanethidine	2 μg/ml		
Hexamethonium	10 μg/ml		
Histamine		100 ng/ml	
Isoprenaline		50 ng/ml	
Leucine-enkephalin		2 ng/ml	125 ng/ml
Methionine-enkephalin		5 ng/ml	250 ng/ml
Morphine		250 ng/ml	
Naloxone		350 ng/ml	
Noradrenaline	2.5 μg/ml	50 ng/ml	1 μg/ml
Papaverine		10 μg/ml	
Phenoxybenzamine			100 ng/ml
Phentolamine		3.5 μg/ml	
Phenylephrine		2 μg/ml	
Propranolol			1 μg/ml
Prostaglandin E$_1$		100 ng/ml	
Tyramine			20 μg/ml

	Guinea-pig	Mouse	Rat
Thymoxamine		300 ng/ml	
Yohimbine		400 pg/ml	

Expt. 5.1 Demonstration of short adrenergic neurones in the guinea-pig vas deferens–hypogastric nerve preparation

The preparation is based on the method of Hukovic (1961). Kill a guinea-pig by dislocating the neck and exsanguinate the animal. Open the abdomen by making a longitudinal cut from the penis up to the rib cage. Lift the gut to one side and raise the terminal end of the colon to expose the hypogastric nerves, which run on either side of the mesentery attached to the colon. Keep

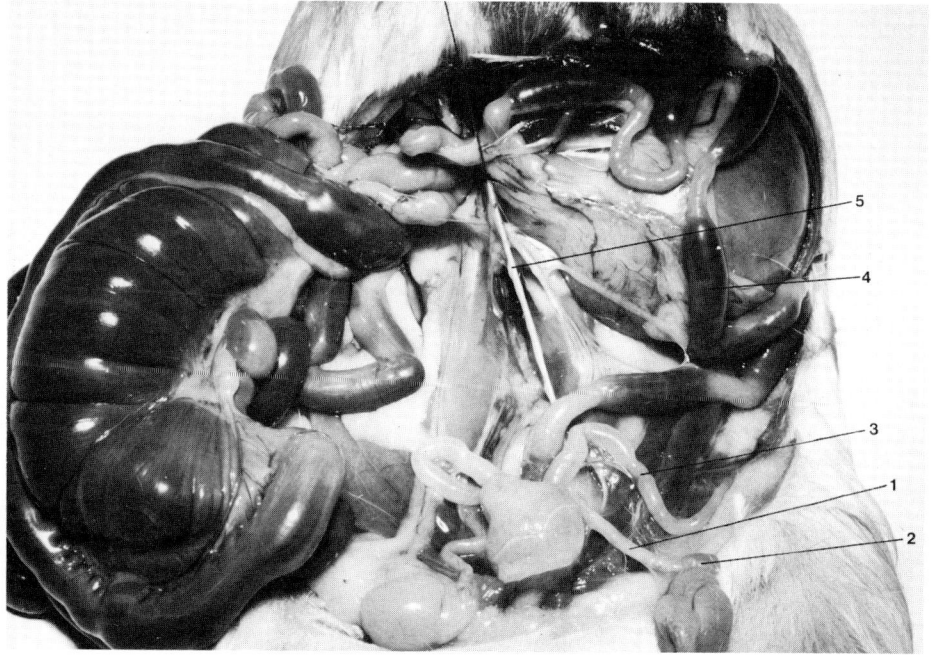

Fig. 25. Dissection of the guinea-pig vas deferens—hypogastric nerve preparation.
The vas deferens (1), is exposed and cut free from the epididymis (2). Do not confuse the vas with the seminal vesicle (3). The terminal colon (4) is pulled to the right hand side and the hypogastric nerves are visible as vary fine structures running in the midline of the abdominal cavity. A tie is placed around the two nerves and they are dissected out together with the surrounding mesentery (5).

the preparation moist at all times with Ringer solution. Insert a threaded needle under both nerves and tie a length of cotton around them at a distance of about 5 cm from the vas deferens. The vas deferens is easily identified as it is white in colour and runs from the epididymis close to the testis to where it joins the urethra. Dissect the nerve back to the vas leaving a substantial amount of mesentery around the muscle where the nerve is very fine and diffuse. Retract the bladder using Spencer Wells forceps and push the testes forward into the abdominal cavity by applying pressure to the scrotum. Both vasa are then free to be dissected. Cut one vas just above the epididymis and carefully dissect the muscle towards the urethra. Free the vas by cutting at the urethra taking care to leave the nervous supply intact where it enters at the urethral end. Free the final portion of the nerve accompanied by a large part of mesentery and transfer the preparation to a petri dish. Both nerve and muscle are delicate, and care must be taken to avoid stretching or handling the tissue excessively with forceps. Tie a thread around the tip of one end of the vas for attachment to the transducer. Tie a second thread around the tip of the other end and attach this to the tissue holder. Transfer the preparation to an organ bath and attach the upper thread to the transducer. Pull the nerve through a Saxby electrode using the attached thread and secure the electrode parallel to the muscle.

Experimental protocol

1 Show frequency-dependent contractions of the vas by carrying out a frequency response curve (5,10,15,20,25,30 Hz). Do not wash the tissue between stimulation.
2 Show two or three dose related submaximal responses with noradrenaline.
3 Choose a frequency which produces a large submaximal response. Show that two or three stimulations at this frequency are constant.
4 Add hexamethonium and without washing repeat 3, followed by a dose of noradrenaline shown to give a submaximal response in 2.
5 If the stimulated response is reduced or abolished wash the preparation and repeat 3 until the stimulated response is constant.
6 Repeat 4 using guanethidine instead of hexamethonium.

The experiment should show that ganglion-blocking drugs reduce the stimulated response indicating that nervous stimulation is pre-ganglionic in origin. In addition, substances which interfere with the release of sympathetic transmitter such as guanethidine also antagonise the nerve-mediated response. If time permits, contractile responses to acetylcholine can also be shown. The lack of effect of atropine on the stimulated response reinforces

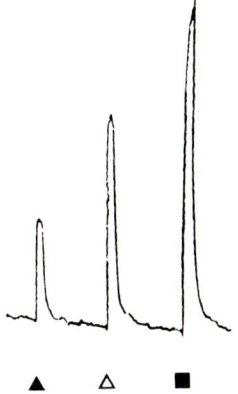

Fig. 26. Responses of the guinea-pig vas hypogastric nerve preparation to direct nerve stimulation (▲ 10 Hz, 10 s; △ 15 Hz, 10 s; ■ 20 Hz, 10 s).

the conclusion that the stimulated response is mediated by the sympathetic branch of the autonomic nervous system.

Expt. 5.2 Opioid agonists and the field-stimulated mouse vas deferens preparation

The preparation is set up based on the methods of Henderson *et al.* (1972) and Hart *et al.* (1979). Kill a mouse by dislocating the neck, open the abdomen and expose the testes and vasa deferentia. The vasa deferentia of the mouse are easily identifiable as white thin tubular structures. Both have blood vessels running along their lengths and they emanate from the epididymis close to the testes. Cut one vas deferens free from the epididymis and dissect it as close to the junction with the urethra as possible. Cut it at this point and transfer it to a petri dish containing Mg^{++}-free Krebs solution. Only a small amount of Krebs is needed to keep the tissue moist and this greatly facilitates the subsequent dissection. Carefully remove all the connective tissue and the blood vessels that closely adhere to the muscle, and expel any semen from the vas by gently pressing the tissue with a finger. Tie a fine thread at the tip of one end of the muscle for attachment to the transducer. Tie another thread around the tip of the other end and secure the preparation to a tissue holder. Transfer the mounted tissue to an organ bath and tie the upper thread to the tranducer.

Experimental protocol

1   Obtain a series of control twitch responses to ensure the stimulated response is constant. Wash the preparation.

2   Stimulate the muscle until the twitch response is constant (usually six control twitches is suitable) and show the inhibitory effect of met-enkephalin.

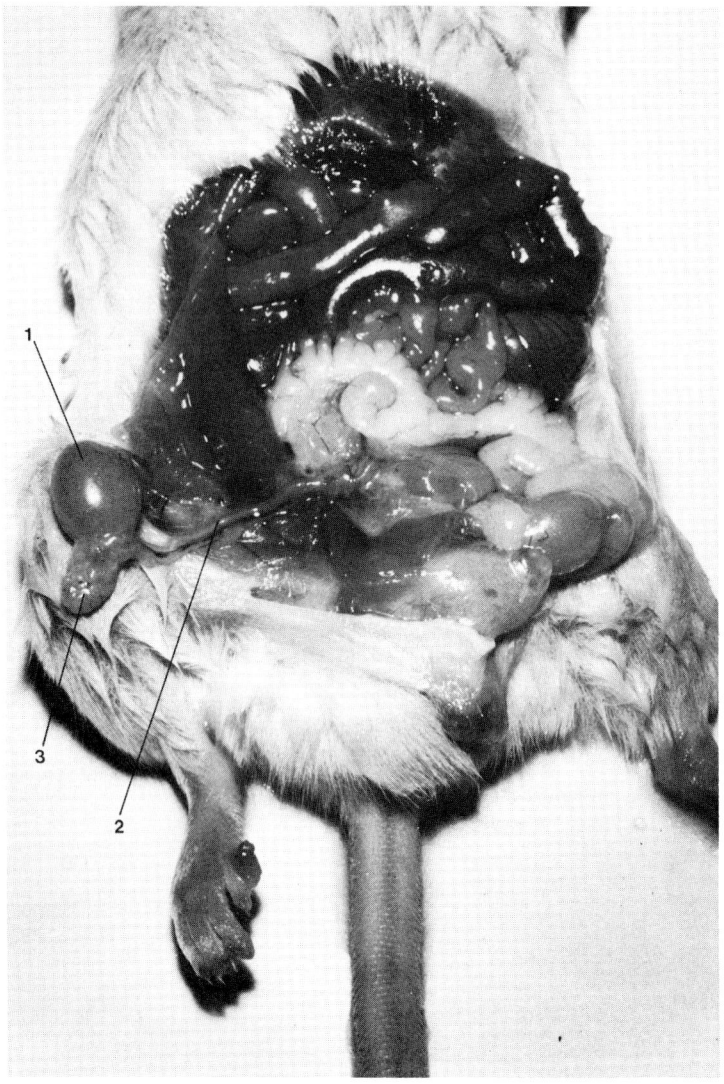

Fig. 27. Dissection of the mouse vas deferens.
The testis (1) is pulled to one side and the vas deferens (2) dissected from the epididymis (3) to where it joins the urethra.

Wash the preparation immediately after maximal twitch height is attained. Carry out a full dose response curve for met-enkephalin allowing 7 minutes between stimulation.

3 Repeat 2 for morphine allowing 10 minutes between doses.

4 Add naloxone to the organ bath and leave in contact with the vas for 15 minutes. Repeat doses of met-enkephalin and morphine that produced maximal inhibitory responses before naloxone.

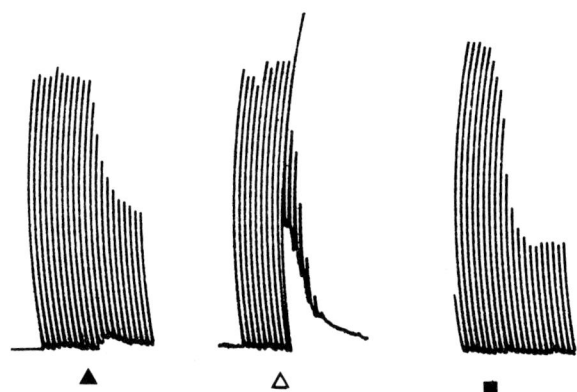

Fig. 28. Responses of the field stimulated mouse vas deferens preparation to noradrenaline (▲ 100 ng/ml, △ 2 µg/ml) and methionine-enkephalin (■ 100 ng/ml).

The experiment should show the qualitative differences between enkephalin and morphine on the vas. The inhibitory response produced by morphine is much slower in onset and offset and morphine is about 30 times less active on the vas. Tachyphylaxis is more commonly observed with morphine and a dose cycle up to 15 minutes may be necessary. Enkephalin is able to produce a total abolition of the twitch response, but the maximal inhibitory effect of morphine is often less than 100% attributed to its partial agonist activity. Naloxone, at a concentration of 350 ng/ml should totally reverse the inhibitory activity of both opioids.

Expt. 5.3 Determination of K_e for naloxone against morphine and met-enkephalin on the field-stimulated mouse vas deferens preparation

Set up the vas as described in Expt. 5.2.

Experimental protocol

1 Carry out full dose response curves for morphine and met-enkephalin as described in Expt. 5.2 ensuring a minimum of three points fall within 20–80% of maximum.

2 Add naloxone (100 ng/ml) to the Ringer reservoir and allow the antagonist to equilibrate with the vas for 20 minutes.

3 Repeat 1 beginning with a concentration of enkephalin 10 times that in 1 and for morphine 100 times that in 1.

It has been usual to express opioid antagonist activity on peripheral isolated tissues as K_e rather than its negative logarithm pA_2, and the principle behind this measure is described on p. 61.

Plot the log-dose response curves for morphine and met-enkephalin before and after antagonist. They should be parallel and the dose ratio can be calculated from the graph comparing the concentrations of agonists which produce the same response in the presence and absence of antagonist. The IC_{50} value is often used for comparison.

$$\text{Dose ratio (DR)} = \frac{A}{a} \frac{\text{(concentration of agonist producing 50\% inhibition of the twitch in the presence of naloxone)}}{\text{(concentration of agonist producing 50\% inhibition of the twitch in the absence of naloxone)}}$$

To increase the accuracy of determination, IC_{50} values should be calculated from linear regression of the log-dose response curves as described on p. 55.

$$K_e = \frac{B \text{ (molar concentration of antagonist)}}{DR - 1}$$

The K_e value for naloxone against morphine is around 2–3 nM whereas the value for met-enkephalin should fall between 20–30 nM. This difference is a reflection of the different opioid receptors which mediate opioid effects in this preparation. Naloxone has a greater selectivity for the μ-receptor through which morphine mediates its effect. Met-enkephalin in contrast is a potent δ-receptor agonist and naloxone is about ten times less effective as an antagonist at this opioid receptor.

Expt. 5.4 Demonstration of pre-synaptic and post-synaptic α-adrenoceptors in the mouse vas deferens

Set up the vas as described in Expt. 5.2.

Experimental protocol

1 Show the effect of clonidine using the protocol described in Expt. 5.2 2.

2 Repeat 1 using phenylephrine.

3 Repeat 1 and 2 adjusting the dose if necessary to show these effects are marked and constant.

4 Add thymoxamine 2 minutes before beginning stimulation. After obtaining stimulated responses (without washing) repeat the dose of clonidine used in 3.

5 Repeat 4 using phenylephrine instead of clonidine.

6 Wash out thymoxamine and repeat 2 until the contractile effect of phenylephrine is restored.

7 Add yohimbine 2 minutes before beginning stimulation. After obtaining stimulated responses (without washing) repeat the dose of phenylephrine used in 3.

8 Repeat 7 using clonidine instead of phenylephrine.

The experiment should show the potentiation of twitch response and contractile activity on the vas of phenylephrine which is mediated via post-synaptic α_1-adrenoceptors. In contrast, clonidine which preferentially stimulates pre-synaptic α_2-adrenoceptors inhibits the release of noradrenaline from the motor nerves and inhibits the twitch response. These two effects can be shown to be distinct by the use of the selective antagonists thymoxamine and yohimbine which block α_1- and α_2-adrenoceptors respectively.

Expt. 5.5 Agonist drugs and the field-stimulated mouse vas deferens preparation

Set up the vas as described in Expt. 5.2.

Experimental protocol

1 Show two or three dose related responses to noradrenaline using the protocol described in Expt. 5.2.2.

2 Show two or three dose related responses to dopamine.

3 Show two or three dose related responses to isoprenaline.

4 Show two or three dose related responses to papaverine.

5 Show two or three dose related responses to morphine.

6 Show two or three dose related responses to ATP.

7 Show two or three dose related responses to prostaglandin E_1.

8 Show two or three dose related responses to histamine.

9 Add naloxone to the Ringer reservoir and repeat a dose of each agonist 1–7 which produced a large submaximal response.

10 Repeat 8 using phentolamine instead of naloxone.

This experiment should show the inhibitory effects of noradrenaline, dopamine, isoprenaline, papaverine, morphine, ATP, prostaglandin E_1 and histamine. Only morphine is antagonised by naloxone and only noradrenaline and dopamine are blocked by the α-adrenoceptor antagonist phentolamine. At high concentrations both dopamine and noradrenaline will contract the vas and phentolamine will antagonise this response by virtue of its post-synaptic α_1-adrenoceptor blocking activity. The experiment can be modified to make a more detailed study of each of these agonists. Inhibitory responses to histamine for example, are mediated via H_2-receptors and blocked by cimetidine. The sensitivity to histamine is strain dependent.

Expt. 5.6 Inhibitory responses of morphine and leu-enkephalin on the field stimulated mouse vas deferens in two different strains of mice

Set up two vas deferens preparations in separate baths as described in Expt. 5.2. One vas should be taken from an albino mouse (preferably BALB/C, T.O. or CD-1 strain), and the second from a black mouse (preferably C57/BL).

Experimental protocol

For both preparations show:

1 A full dose response curve to morphine.

2 A full dose response curve to leu-enkephalin.

Calculate the IC_{50} value for morphine and leu-enkephalin (i.e. the concentration of agonist producing 50% inhibition of the twitch responses) using linear regression of points between 20% and 80% of maximum.

The experiment should show the disparity in sensitivity of different strains of mice to the two opioid agonists. Most albino strains have both μ- and predominantly δ-receptors and both morphine (a μ-receptor agonist) and leu-enkephalin (a δ-receptor agonist) inhibit the vas. The relative potency is in the order of 15-fold in favour of leu-enkephalin. In contrast C57 black mice have virtually no μ-receptors and are extremely insensitive to morphine. If an IC_{50} value can be computed, the relative potency is often 100-fold in favour of leu-enkephalin.

Expt. 5.7 Effect of peptidase inhibition on opioid peptide activity on the field stimulated rat vas deferens preparation

Set up the rat vas deferens as described for the mouse in Expt. 5.2.

Experimental protocol

1 Obtain a series of control twitch responses to ensure the stimulated response is constant. Wash the preparation.
2 Carry out a full dose response curve to met-enkephalin as described in Expt. 5.2 2.
3 Repeat 2 for leu-enkephalin.
4 Repeat 3 for (D-Ala^2, D-Leu^5)-enkephalin.
5 Add leucyl-leucine (300 μg/ml) to the Krebs and allow to equilibrate for ten minutes.
6 Repeat 2 starting with a 30-fold lower dose.
7 Repeat 3 starting with a 20-fold lower dose.
8 Repeat 4.

This experiment should show the increase in potency of the enkephalin pentapeptides by use of leucyl-leucine which presumably acts by substrate inhibition of peptidase enzymes. In contrast the stable enkephalin analogue is no more active in the presence of leucyl-leucine. A further increase in activity of met- and leu-enkephalin (up to 200-fold) can be achieved by including the aminopeptidase inhibitor bestatin (3.5μg/ml) in the Krebs medium. The cost of this compound is however often prohibitive.

Expt. 5.8 Indirectly-acting sympathomimetics and the field stimulated rat vas deferens preparation

Set up the rat vas deferens as described in Expt. 5.7. Include propranolol and atropine in the Krebs ringer.

Experimental protocol

1 Obtain a series of control twitch responses to ensure the stimulated response is constant. Momentarily cease stimulation and without washing show the effect of noradrenaline.

2 Repeat 1 using tyramine instead of noradrenaline and leave in contact with the preparation for 4 minutes. Without washing stimulate the tissue for a further 2 minutes.

3 Show the effect of two or three doses of cocaine on field-stimulated responses.

4 Add phenoxybenzamine to the Ringer reservoir and repeat 1 2 and 3.

Both tyramine and noradrenaline should contract the rat vas, an effect blocked by phenoxybenzamine. The inhibitory pre-synaptic effect of tyramine and cocaine on the field-stimulated responses should be unaffected by phenoxybenzamine. Propranolol and atropine are included in the Ringer to exclude interactions at β-adrenoceptors or muscarinic receptors respectively.

Cardiac and Vascular Preparations

Introduction

Cardiac preparations

The heart is innervated by both sympathetic and parasympathetic nerves. This innervation alters the basic rhythm of the heart that is initiated by the pacemaker tissue of the SA node. When the heart is removed from the intact animal and maintained in an isolated system, the heart will beat spontaneously by virtue of the myogenic rhythm controlled by the SA node. The parasympathetic supply arises from vagal axons which supply the SA node, atrial muscle, AV node and bundle. It is generally believed that parasympathetic nerves do not supply the ventricles, and there are no muscarinic receptors in ventricular muscle. Though there is some controversy as to whether sympathetic nerves directly innervate the ventricles, noradrenaline released from sympathetic nerves reaches the ventricles and β_1- and few β_2-adrenoceptors are present in ventricular muscle. Stimulation of the sympathetic supply produces both positive inotropic (increase in force) and chronotropic (increase in rate) effects. Stimulation of parasympathetic nerves and release of acetylcholine produces negative chronotropic (decrease in rate) effects. In addition, acetylcholine has a direct negative inotropic effect (decrease in force) on the atrial myocardium.

The negative chronotropic and inotropic effects of acetylcholine can be demonstrated in isolated preparations of separated right and left atria and this is shown in Expt. 6.4. The right atrium containing the SA node beats spontaneously. Rabbit or guinea-pig atria can be used.

Blood is supplied to the walls of the heart by the coronary arteries. Postganglionic sympathetic axons pass from the main cardiac sympathetic nerves to the coronary vessels. There is no parasympathetic innervation of the vascular supply to the heart. It is probable that α-adrenoceptors mediating vasoconstriction are present in the large coronary arteries and β_2-adrenoceptors mediating vasodilation exist in the smaller vessels. However, coronary blood vessels are very sensitive to vasodilator metabolites released from the myocardial cells, especially under hypoxic conditions. This effect probably predominates in isolated preparations.

Isolated rabbit, rat or guinea-pig hearts can be maintained by perfusing the coronary arteries using the method of Langendorff (1895). The aorta is cannulated and the technique is therefore a retrograde perfusion. The pressure of Ringer solution closes the aortic valve so that the Ringer is delivered directly to the mouths of the coronary arteries without passing through the heart. The aortic valves prevent the left ventricle from filling, and the left side of the heart remains empty. The right side receives the fluid draining from the coronary sinus and this is expelled through the cut orifices of the inferior venae cavae or passes through the right ventricle and is pumped out of the cut pulmonary artery. In the isolated heart the muscle is doing very little work and there is no real cardiac output. The rate at which fluid leaves the heart reflects the coronary flow, and will continue even if the heart is dead. An isolated heart, perfused as described, will beat myogenically and the force of ventricular contraction can be measured by attaching a thread from the tip of the ventricles through a pulley system to a transducer. Using a tachograph pre-amplifier the heart rate can be integrated from the trace of ventricular contraction. The tachograph times the interval between contractions and relaxations from two pre-set trigger points and integrates a rate from this information (Fig. 5, p. 19). In addition to measuring force and rate, it is possible to record coronary resistance if the flow rate is constantly maintained by a peristaltic pump and a pressure transducer is placed between the pump and the heart. This is a relatively poor indicator, since vessels are mostly maximally dilated.

Guinea-pig or rat hearts are usually perfused with Krebs solution, but rabbit hearts do better with McEwens solution which has added sucrose in order to increase the osmotic pressure. The oxygen requirement of cardiac muscle is high and it is important to saturate the Ringer solution with oxygen. Isolated hearts often work best if they are plunged into ice-cold Ringer immediately after removing from the animal. This arrests movement of the beating heart, thereby reducing the requirements for glucose and oxygen. The lack of movement also makes it easier to remove any clots and cannulate the preparation. After setting up the preparation, the perfusion temperature should be raised from room temperature. If the heart is exposed immediately to 37°C, rhythm disorders are often observed. The rabbit heart will go on beating for 9 hours if not insulted by toxic drugs.

Vascular preparations

In contrast to the heart, blood vessels are served almost exclusively by the sympathetic branch of the autonomic nervous system. The distribution of adrenoceptors at the post-synaptic terminals of vasomotor nerves, varies considerably from tissue to tissue. α-adrenoceptors mediate vasoconstriction and there is a predominance of these receptors in blood vessels serving the skin and viscera. β-adrenoceptors (mostly of the β_2 type) mediate vasodilation and predominate in skeletal muscle blood vessels. A few blood vessels are served by cholinergic sympathetic nerves and there are probably some dopaminergic vasodilator nerves. Arteries also possess isolated muscarinic receptors which are devoid of innervation. These receptors mediate vasodilation and this can be observed in response to cholinergic agonists.

In order to study *in vitro* constriction of blood vessels in response to drugs, it is necessary to cut spiral strips of arteries. The movement of circular muscle can therefore be measured in a longitudinal plane. The aortic strip is a suitable preparation (Expt. 6.5), and possesses mixed α- and β_2-receptors as well as isolated muscarinic receptors. One can never be sure, using spirally cut strips, that the response of such a preparation reflects what occurs normally (for example, acetylcholine causes contraction of strip preparations whereas *in vivo* it produces relaxation). Also the responses of large arteries may not be typical of the vascular tree as a whole. Perfused vascular beds, e.g. rabbit ear and rat hind quarters have been useful, but oedema of the tissues induced by perfusion with fluids with no colloidal osmotic pressure restrict the use of such preparations. One of the more useful preparations is the perfused mesenteric vessels of the rat (Expt. 6.6) and reflects more closely, the true action of drugs on the vascular system. A great advantage of this preparation is that the sympathetic nerve supply to the vascular bed can be stimulated merely by placing electrodes around the mesenteric artery, just distal to the point of cannulation, since the sympathetic nerves run together with the arteries.

Drugs

Sympathomimetics

Adrenaline, noradrenaline and isoprenaline stimulate the myocardium directly causing positive inotropic and chronotropic effects. These effects are mediated via β_1-adrenoceptors and can be blocked by β-adrenoceptor antagonists such as propranolol. Both noradrenaline and isoprenaline often produce dysrhythmias and this can be observed in the isolated heart. Isoprenaline is about ten times more potent in stimulating the heart than adrenaline or noradrenaline and its effects are often more prolonged. This, in part, may reflect the lack of reuptake of this amine. All three amines in isolated preparations dilate the coronary vessels though the direct effect on the vessels is probably vasoconstriction. In the isolated heart preparations, the vessels are often maximally dilated and any effect is therefore masked.

In the isolated aortic strip preparation, both adrenaline and noradrenaline produce contraction. In perfused vascular bed preparations, their vasoconstrictor activity can be demonstrated. These effects are mediated via α-adrenoceptors and are unaffected by propranolol but antagonised by the α-adrenoceptor blocking drug phentolamine.

Cholinomimetics

Drugs which stimulate muscarinic receptors produce negative chronotropic effects and sometimes negative inotropic effects. If large enough doses of acetylcholine are given, the heart will stop beating (though the coronary flow will still continue). The heart can be restarted by using high doses of atropine to competitively displace acetylcholine from its muscarinic sites.

Cholinomimetics are often ineffective in vascular strip preparations or produce anomolous contractile responses. In vascular bed preparations, the vessels are often maximally dilated and the dilating effect of acetylcholine can only be demonstrated by showing physiological antagonism of, for example, the vasoconstrictor effect of noradrenaline.

Angiotensin and Vasopressin

Angiotensin II is the most potent pressor substance known, and produces marked vasconstriction in vascular bed preparations. Its constrictor activity in coronary arterioles is probably relatively less than in arterioles elsewhere and vasopressin is a more suitable vasoconstrictor to show the effect on coronary vessels in isolated heart preparations. Both the effect on angiotensin II and vasopressin are mediated by a direct action on the smooth muscle of the vessels.

Nitrites

Nitrites dilate coronary vessels but in perfused isolated heart preparations these vessels are often maximally dilated. However, if nitrites are given after vasconstriction by an agent such as vasopressin the dilator effect may be observed.

Xanthines

Caffeine, theophylline and xanthine derivatives are peripheral vasodilators. They produce mild stimulation of the heart muscle but this effect is species dependent. Guinea-pig and rat hearts show this action, but is rarely seen in the isolated rabbit heart.

Anaesthetics

Chloroform and ether both depress the cardiac muscle. The doses of modern anaesthetics employed for operative procedures do not produce these effects. The major disadvantage of chloroform is to sensitise the heart muscle to the dysrhythmia-inducing properties of aderenaline.

Dysrhythmics and antidysrhythmics

The alkaloid aconitine, when placed on the surface of the exposed heart, causes an ectopic focus and generation of cardiac dysrhythmias. It delays repolarisation of conducting fibre action potentials which outlast the refractory period, and the resultant after-potentials trigger dysrhythmic activity. The surface of the isolated perfused heart is continuously washed with leaking fluid, so the application to the surface is impractical. However, if tincture of aconite is injected slowly an acceleration of heartbeat is observed and an ectopic focus deep in the tip of the ventricles is generated leading to ventricular tachycardia. A wave of contraction spreading upwards from the apex of the ventricles can be observed by handling the heart. The surface sometimes may seem to have a rolling motion. The efficient pumping movement is lost, the atria contract after the ventricles (retrograde conduction in the Bundle of His) and often fail to respond to every ventricular beat. Ventricular tachycardia and fibrillation can be reversed by antidysrhythmic drugs such as lignocaine. it prolongs the effective refractory period (i.e. the ratio of refractory period to action potential duration) of heart muscle by stabilising the cell membranes, but without depressing the resting potential significantly.

Histamine

Histamine causes constriction of coronary vessels mediated by H_1-receptors and blocked by mepyramine. Dilation, mediated by H_2-receptors, is sometimes observed when the H_1-receptors are blocked. In the isolated heart, histamine has a positive inotropic and chronotropic effect. It is mediated by H_2-receptors and can be blocked by cimetidine. Part of this effect may depend on the release of noradrenaline from sympathetic nerves.

Experimental parameters

Organ bath	Rabbit heart	Open 100 ml chamber
	Rat heart	Open 50 ml chamber
	Guinea-pig atria	20 ml
	Rabbit aortic strip	20 ml
	Rat mesenteric vessels	Open 50 ml horizontal chamber
Ringer solution	Rabbit heart	McEwens
	Rat heart	Krebs
	Guinea-pig atria	Krebs or Ringer Locke
	Rabbit aortic strip	Krebs
	Rat mesenteric vessels	Krebs
Aeration	McEwens and Krebs	95% O_2 5% CO_2
	Ringer Locke	O_2
Bath temperature	Isolated heart	37°C
	Isolated atria	30°C
	Isolated aorta	37°C
	Mesenteric vessels	37°C
Recording	Isolated heart/atria	Isometric
	Aortic strip	Isotonic
	Mesenteric vessels	Pressure
Resting tension	Rabbit heart	3–4 g
	Rat heart	2–3 g
	Guinea-pig atria	1 g
	Rabbit aortic strip	2–3 g
Equilibration period		45 minutes
Dose cycle	Isolated heart	2–5 minutes
	Guinea-pig atria	6 minutes
	Rabbit aortic strip	7 minutes
	Rat mesenteric vessels	3–5 minutes
Contact time	Guinea-pig atria	1 minute
	Rabbit aortic strip	2–3 minutes
Stimulus parameters	Expt. 6.7	Pulse width 5 ms
		Voltage 15–30 V
		Frequency 5–50 Hz
		Stimulus duration 30 s

Drugs (final concentration: starting dose)

	Rabbit and rat heart	Guinea-pig atria	Rabbit aortic strip	Rat mesenteric vessels
Acetylcholine	400 ng		250 ng/ml	
Adrenaline	200 ng		100 ng/ml	100 ng
Angiotensin II				10 ng
Atropine	20 μg			
Cocaine			200 ng/ml	
Guanethidine				1 μg/ml
Histamine	200 ng			
Isoprenaline	20 ng	5 ng/ml	50 ng/ml	
Noradrenaline	200 ng		100 ng/ml	100 ng
Phentolamine				1 μg/ml
Practololol		150 ng/ml		
Propranolol	50 μg	150 ng/ml		1 μg/ml
Salbutamol		2.5 μg/ml		
Sodium nitrite	500 μg			
Vasopressin	0.05 U			0.01 U

Expt. 6.1 Drugs and the isolated rabbit heart

Before beginning the experiment it is important to ensure that the perfusion apparatus is primed and the Ringer solution has been saturated with 95% O_2/ 5% CO_2. If a detachable cannula system is used, ensure that this is full of ice-cold Ringer. The cannula should have a side arm for drug administration and for flushing the system with Ringer solution.

The isolated heart is set up based on the methid of Langendorff (1895). Kill a rabbit by dislocating the neck and exsanguinate the animal. Open the thorax immediately, expose and remove the heart as rapidly as possible and plunge the tissue into ice-cold McEwen's solution. Ensure that at least 1 cm of aorta is removed intact. Do not worry about carefully trimming lung tissue away from the heart as this can be done at a later stage. Squeeze the heart firmly to expel blood from the organ and prevent the formation of clots. Remove the heart from the Ringer solution and examine the major veins and arteries to ensure no clots are present. Remove any clotted blood with fine forceps. Trip away any excess connective and lung tissue from the heart taking care not to damage the atria. Re-immerse the heart in ice-cold Ringer and squeeze the ventricles again. Remove the heart and locate the aorta. If a detachable cannula is used (and in the author's view this is preferable) locate the cannula tip about 0.5 cm into the aorta and tie firmly in place with button thread. Secure the thread around the side arm of the cannula to ensure that the perfusion pressure of the heart does not push it off. Return the mounted heart to the ice-cold Ringer and squeeze the tissue to ensure no air bubbles are present. It is important to exclude air from the perfusion system otherwise air emboli will be formed. Transfer the heart to the perfusion apparatus and begin perfusing immediately. When a detachable cannula is not available it will be necessary to tie the heart to the cannula attached to the perfusion system. This usually requires two pairs of hands and care must be taken to exclude air bubbles. Initially flush the side arm with Ringer and then close this off and perfuse the coronary vessels. Begin with a high perfusion pressure. If a constant head reservoir system is used for providing pressure, raise this to about 3 feet above the cannula for 1–2 minutes before locating the reservoir about 18″ above the level of the heart. Alternatively, if a peristaltic pump is used set the rate for about 15–20 ml per minute reducing to 3–5 ml per minute. Switch on the water circulator to raise the perfusion chamber and Ringer temperature to 37°C. Gas bubbles may form in the warming coil and it is best to have a gas trap device in the perfusion system to prevent air embolism. Two methods are proposed. The first utilises an inverted tube located in line with the perfusion medium and connected by a T-piece. The tube is filled with the perfusing medium. Air bubbles are displaced into this tube and as the experiment progresses the Ringer level in the trap falls. The second method involves the use of a three-arm cannula with a rubber diaphragm inserted over the upper arm. Gas is vented through a fine needle inserted into the diaphragm (Fig. 29). Drugs can also be given using this needle.

Attach a heart clip complete with a length of thread to the tip of the ventricles. Locate the thread around a pulley about 4 cm vertically below the heart. Attach the thread to the transducer after locating over a second pulley horizontal to the first and about 20 cm apart (Fig. 29). In order to maintain the air temperature around the heart close to 37°C it is usually surrounded by a water jacket maintained at this temperature. Drug additions should be made by attaching a syringe to the injection port which should have a luer fitting tip and drug volumes should be kept to <0.2 ml. Adequate time for recovery should be allowed between each dose, and before each drug addition the heart rate should be steady.

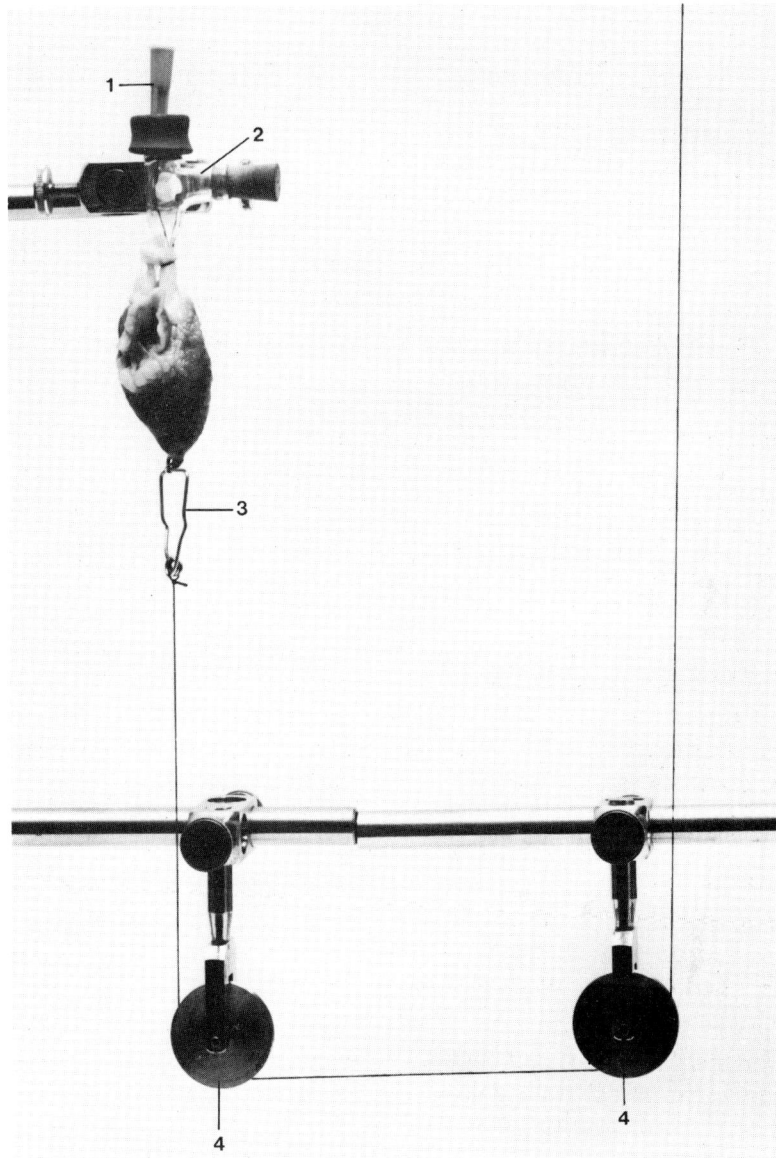

Fig. 29. Perfused heart apparatus.

Perfusion fluid passes through the coronary vessels via the three arm cannula (2). Air bubbles are vented via the needle (1) and drugs can be administered by this route. A heart clip (3) is attached to the tip of the ventricles and the thread run over two pulleys (4) for attachment to the transducer.

Experimental protocol

Show the effect of 0.2 ml of the following drugs. If the response is not marked, double the dose.

1   0.2 ml 0.9% saline (this should produce no effect).
2   Adrenaline.
3   Noradrenaline.
4   Isoprenaline.
5   Chloroform 1 in 500 0.5 ml.
6   Acetylcholine.
7   Acetylcholine (40 μg). When the heart has stoped beating for 3–4 seconds add atropine. When the heart re-starts repeat acetylcholine.
8   Repeat 2, 3 and 4. When the effect of isoprenaline is approaching maximum add propranolol.
9   Repeat 2, 3 and 4.
10 Count the drops of fluid leaving the heart for a control period of 15 seconds. Add vasopressin and count the drops for two periods of 15 seconds starting 5 seconds after the vasopressin is injected.
11 Repeat 10 using sodium nitrite instead of vasopressin.

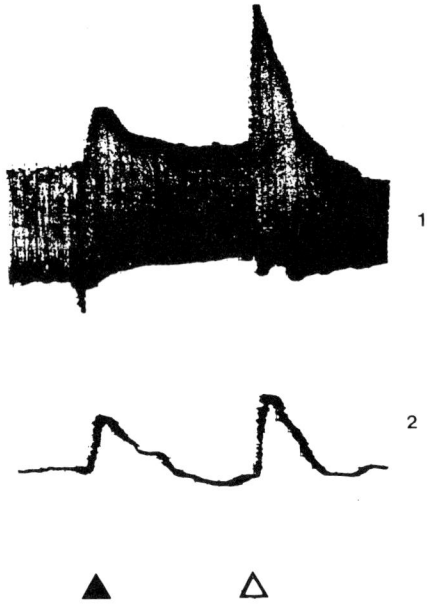

Fig. 30. Responses of the isolated rabbit heart to noradrenaline (▲ 200 ng, △ 1 μg).
1 Inotropic effects.
2 Chrontropic effects.

12 Add tincture of aconite (0.2 ml) slowly over one minute until dysrhythmia develops. Handle the heart to observe this effect.

13 Add lignocaine (2%) very slowly. Sufficient lignocaine should be added to just produce standstill of the heart. When the beat recommences examine and handle the heart, and repeat if necessary until normal rhythm is re-established.

This experiment should demonstrate the effects of drugs on heart force and rate described in the introduction to this section. In addition, constriction of coronary arteries as evidenced by a decrease in flow rate may be observed and it is possible to induce disorders of rhythm and reverse dysrhythmia in the isolated heart.

Expt. 6.2 The action of histamine on the isolated rabbit heart

Set up the heart as described in Expt. 6.1 with the following modification. Perfuse the preparation by means of a peristaltic pump. After initial perfusion at a rapid rate, decrease the pump speed so that the coronary vessels are perfused at the minimum rate that will support a constant rate and force of beat. In addition, the apparatus should have a pressure transducer connected to a side arm between the pump and the heart for measurement of coronary resistance.

Experimental protocol

Use 0.2 ml for all the drugs injected.

1 Show the effect of noradrenaline and adrenaline.

2 Show the effect of increasing doses of histamine (up to 20 μg).

3 Add propranolol (1 μg/ml) to the perfusion fluid reservoir and repeat 1 and a dose of histamine which produces an effect on the heart.

4 Add mepyramine (5 μg/ml) to the perfusion fluid reservoir and repeat the dose of histamine used in 3.

5 Add cimetidine (2.5 μg/ml) to the perfusion fluid reservoir and repeat the dose of histamine used in 4.

This experiment should show that the positive inotropic and chronotropic effects of histamine on the heart are unaffected by a high dose of mepyramine but blocked by the H_2-antagonist cimetidine. It may be possible to observe an increase in coronary resistance which is blocked by mepyramine, and also that the inotropic and chronotropic effects are slightly reduced by a dose of propranolol which blocks the actions of noradrenaline and adrenaline.

Expt. 6.3 Effects of acetylcholine on the atropinised isolated rat heart preparation

Set up an isolated rat heart using the method described for the rabbit in Expt. 6.1. The aorta of the rat heart is easily identifiable by its opaque white appearance. In contrast, the other major arteries and veins are a silvery white colour.

Experimental protocol

Use 0.2 ml for all the drugs injected.
1 Show the effect of two or three doses of noradrenaline, adrenaline and acetylcholine.
2 Add atropine (1 μg/ml) to the perfusion fluid reservoir and allow 15 minutes for equilibration with the antagonist.
3 Repeat acetylcholine increasing the dose until an effect on the heart is observed.
4 Repeat noradrenaline and adrenaline.
5 Add propranolol (1 μg/ml) to the perfusion fluid reservoir in addition to atropine.
6 Repeat the dose of acetylcholine which produced a response in 3 and the dose of noradrenaline and adrenaline that produced a response in 4.

This experiment should show that acetylcholine can produce an adrenergic-like effect if its muscarinic effects are blocked by atropine. This effect manifested as a positive inotropic and chronotropic effect is like noradrenaline and adrenaline, blocked by propanolol. The mechanism underlying this effect of acetylcholine is still a matter of controversy, though it is probable that it results from release of noradrenaline from sympathetic nerves, and is mediated by nicotinic receptors at the nerve terminal.

Expt. 6.4 The nature of adrenoceptors in the isolated guinea-pig atria preparation

Kill a large guinea-pig by dislocating its neck and exsanguinate the animal. Remove the heart as described in Expt. 6.1, and after removing the blood, transfer the heart to a petri dish containing ice-cold aerated Ringer solution. Remove the pericardium and fat carefully. Dissect off the ventricles taking care not to cut into the atria so as not to damage the pacemaker. Tie threads to the tip of each atrium and mount the preparation on a tissue holder.

Transfer the tissue to an organ bath and attach the upper thread to a transducer.

Experimental protocol

1 Add isoprenaline.
2 Add salbutamol.
3 Add practolol 3 minutes before repeating 1.
4 Add practolol 3 minutes before repeating 2.
5 Repeat 1 and 2 until the original responses are restored.
6 Repeat 3 and 4 using propranolol instead of practolol.

This experiment should demonstrate the presence (albeit a minor proportion) of β_2-adrenoceptors in atria. Usually the responses to isoprenaline and especially salbutamol are not totally blocked by practolol which is selective for β_1-adrenoceptors. Propranolol which blocks both β_1- and β_2-adrenoceptors abolishes responses to isoprenaline and salbutamol.

Expt. 6.5 Drugs and the rabbit aortic strip preparation

The preparation is based on the method of Furchgott and Bhadrakom (1953). Kill a rabbit by a blow on the neck and exsanguinate the animal. Open the chest and pull the internal viscera to one side exposing the aorta. Cut the aorta close to the heart and dissect out the aorta as far as possible. Several strip preparations can be made from one rabbit. Transfer the tissue to a petri dish containing aerated Ringer solution and divide the aorta into 3–4 cm lengths. Locate the aorta over a large serum needle or thin glass rod to facilitate preparation of a strip of tissue. Remove any surrounding fat or connective tissue and then cut the aorta spirally, so as to produce a continuous strip. Curved scissors are often useful for this procedure. Tie a thread to each end of the strip and attach one end to the tissue holder. Transfer the mounted tissue to an organ bath and attach the upper thread to the transducer.

Experimental protocol

1 Show dose related effects to noradrenaline and adrenaline.
2 Choose a dose of noradrenaline which gives a large submaximal response. Add cocaine followed 1 minute later, without washing, by the noradrenaline dose.
3 Repeat noradrenaline until the response returns to the original level.

4 Repeat 2 and 3 for adrenaline instead of noradrenaline.

5 Add isoprenaline and repeat the dose of adrenaline used in 4. If the response to adrenaline is not reduced repeat using a larger dose of isoprenaline.

6 Repeat adrenaline until the response returns to the original level.

7 Repeat 5 using acetylcholine instead of isoprenaline.

This experiment should show the contractile effect of noradrenaline and adrenaline on this vascular strip. Noradrenaline should be potentiated to a greater extent than adrenaline by cocaine (which blocks Uptake I) since it has a higher affinity for this uptake mechanism. Both acetylcholine and isoprena-

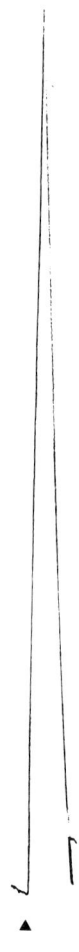

Fig. 31. Response of the rabbit aortic strip to
adrenaline (▲ 75 pg/ml).

line sometimes produce contraction of the strip mediated via muscarinic and α-adrenoceptors respectively. However it is possible to observe relaxation which is the expected response (that of isoprenaline being mediated by β_2-adrenoceptors) and it is then possible to show physiological antagonism of the α-mediated contraction, induced by adrenaline.

Expt. 6.6 Drugs and the perfused mesenteric vessels of the rat

The preparation is based on the method of McGregor (1965). Anaesthetise a rat by exposing the animal to ether in a sealed box. Remove the rat and maintain the ether anaesthesia by means of ether soaked cotton wool held in a small beaker and placed close to the animals snout. Sodium pentobarbitone (6 mg/100 g i.p.) can be used as an alternative anaesthetic. Open the abdomen and locate the aorta and the superior (anterior) mesenteric artery. This artery lies between the coeliac artery and the left renal artery and vein and is virtually opposite the right kidney. The artery passes diagonally downwards from the aorta towards the right side of the animal. Clear the vessels and place two threads underneath the mesenteric artery. If you wish you may tie off the large branches of this artery which serve the duodenum and pancreas but the preparation will work adequately without doing this as long as the cannula is inserted a sufficient distance into the artery. Keep the vessel and mesentery moist at all times with 0.9% saline. Using one thread make a tie at the aortic end of the mesenteric artery. Using fine pointed scissors make an incision in the artery and with the aid of fine iris forceps insert a polythene cannula (0.75 mm external diameter) about 2.5 cm into the vessel. Make sure the cannula is primed with 0.9% saline and connected to a full 5 ml syringe. Tie in the cannula with the second thread. Remove the mesentery from the intestine beginning from the lowest point of attachment, cutting as close as possible to the intestinal border of the mesentery. Final remove any connective tissue still attached to the artery and free the vessel and mesentery from the animal. Kill the rat by dislocating the neck. Flush the vascular system with 0.9% saline and then attach the cannula to a three way tap connected to a perfusion apparatus containing Krebs ringer. Place the preparation in an open-ended organ bath positioned horizontally instead of vertically thereby surrounding the tissue with a heated water jacket. Perfuse the arterial tree with Krebs at a rate of 2–10 ml/min using a peristaltic pump. A pressure transducer is connected between the pump and the preparation, similarly to that described for measuring coronary resistance in Expt. 6.3. Administer drugs by means of a

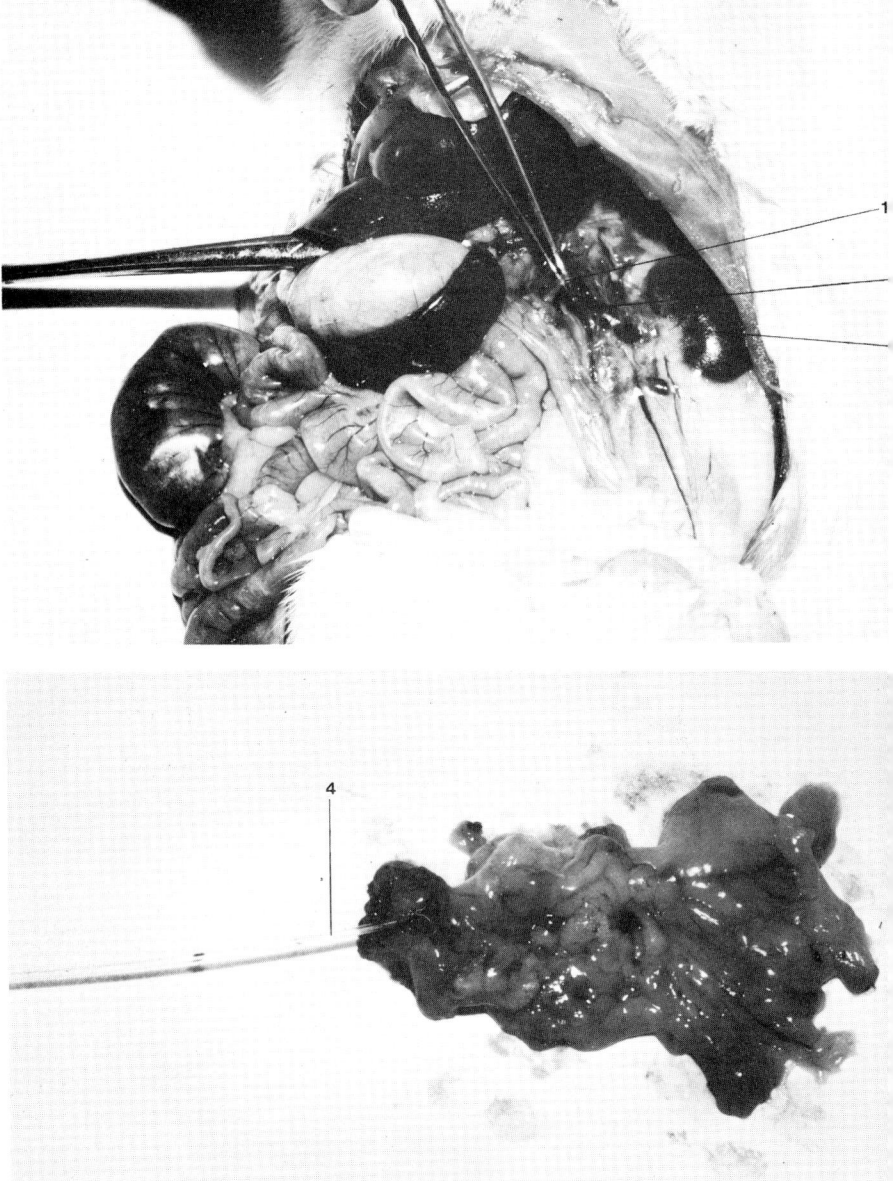

Fig. 32. Dissection of the isolated mesenteric vessels of the rat.

The intestine is pulled to one side and the superior mesenteric artery (1) is prepared for cannulation. The inferior vena cava (2) and right kidney (3) are useful guides to locating this artery. A cannula (4) is inserted into the artery and the mesentery removed from the intestine to produce the isolated preparation.

syringe connected to the three way tap. Allow some perfusion fluid to rinse out the dead space in the tap between each injection.

Experimental protocol

1   Inject adrenaline and show two or three dose related responses.
2   Repeat 1 for noradrenaline.
3   Repeat 1 for angiotensin II.
4   Repeat 1 for vasopressin.
5   Add propranolol to the Krebs perfusion fluid and perfuse the vascular bed for 10 minutes. Repeat doses of 1–4 which produced a large submaximal response.
6   Repeat 5 using phentolamine in addition to the propranolol.

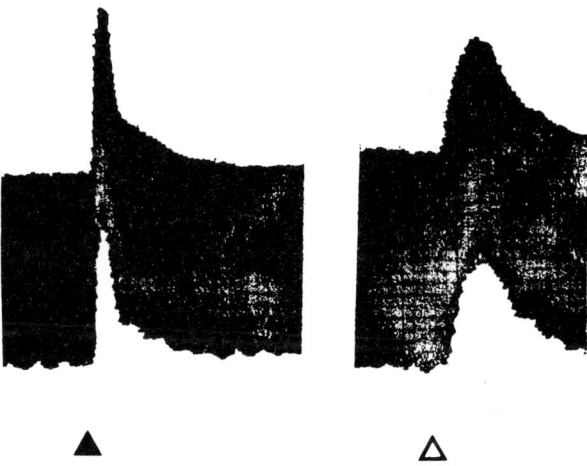

Fig. 33. Responses of the isolated perfused mesenteric vessels of the rat to adrenaline (▲ 4 μg) and vasopressin (△ 20 mU).

This experiment should demonstrate the vasoconstrictor activity of adrenaline, noradrenaline, angiotensin and vasopressin. The effects of noradrenaline and adrenaline are mediated via α-adrenoceptors and blocked by phentolamine. Part of the vasoconstrictor activity of angiotensin may be mediated via noradrenaline release and phentolamine may partially antagonise angiotensin responses.

Expt. 6.7 Effect of drugs on nerve-stimulated responses of the perfused mesenteric vessels of the rat

Set up the perfused mesenteric preparation as described in Expt. 6.6. In addition secure hook or jaw electrodes around the mesenteric artery just distal to the cannula.

Experimental protocol

1 Show two or three dose related responses to noradrenaline.
2 Show frequency related responses between 5 and 50 Hz.
3 Add guanethidine to the Krebs perfusion fluid and perfuse the vascular bed for 10 minutes.
4 Repeat 1.
5 Repeat 2.

The experiment should demonstrate that the nerve mediated responses are sympathetic in origin, and blocked by an adrenergic neurone blocker such as guanethidine. Sensitivity to agonists acting upon post-synaptic adrenoceptors is unaffected (cf. Expt. 2.4). The effects of stimulation can enhance exogenous noradrenaline responses and this may be observed when repeating noradrenaline doses after electrical stimulation.

Isolated Stomach

Introduction

The stomach can be divided into three sections. The upper part of the stomach is the fundus, the main body is known as the corpus and the aboral end is the pyloric portion. In the rat the external appearance indicates only two clear portions, an upper grey area which is the fundal region and a lower pink area often referred to as the pyloric region. The fundus usually contains swallowed air and its function appears to be primarily concerned with pressure changes. Movements of the circular muscle of the fundal region can be measured in a longitudinal plane by preparing a strip preparation of the muscle and this is shown in Expt. 7.1 and 7.2. The contraction observed in this tissue is often well-maintained and a stretching weight is often required to bring the response back to the baseline.

Drugs

Autacoids

Despite the large amounts of histamine and histidine decarboxylase in the rat stomach the fundal strip preparation is relatively insensitive to histamine. There appear to be few H_1 receptors in the muscle.

In contrast, the rat fundus is extremely sensitive to 5-hydroxytryptamine and at one time was used as a bioassay preparation for the amine. The metabolism of 5-hydroxytryptamine *in vivo* is primarily effected by the enzyme monoamine oxidase. However, in this isolated tissue preparation monoamine oxidase inhibitor drugs are usually unable to potentiate 5-hydroxytryptamine responses unlike the anticholinesterase potentiation of acetylcholine responses. This may be due to the fact that monoamine oxidase is a mitochondrial enzyme and despite its high concentration in the stomach it may not have access to 5-hydroxytryptamine. This hypothesis is supported by the observation that tryptamine which is a less polar agonist is potentiated by monoamine oxidase inhibitors. The effects of monoamine oxidase inhibitors on

5-hydroxytryptamine and tryptamine responses is shown in Expt. 7.2 Unlike isolated intestinal preparations the responses to 5-hydroxytryptamine are mediated predominantly via D-receptors (see p. 42).

Bradykinin is a powerful stimulant of isolated intestinal preparations and produces a characteristic slow contraction of fundal strips. This is a direct effect on the smooth muscle and is not antagonised by atropine, H_1-blockers or ganglion blocking drugs.

Cholinomimetics

Like intestinal muscle all muscarinic agonists cause contraction of fundal strips, and the responses are blocked by atropine.

Experimental parameters

Organ bath	20 ml
Ringer solution	Krebs
Aeration	95% O_2/5% CO_2
Bath temperature	32°C/37°C
Recording	Isotonic
Resting tension	1 g (+ 1 g streching weight)
Equilibration period	45–60 minutes
Dose cycle	6 minutes
Contact time	1–2 minutes

Drugs (final bath concentration—starting dose)

Acetylcholine	25 ng/ml
Bradykinin	500 pg/ml
Bromolysergic acid diethylamide	1 μg/ml
Histamine	5 μg/ml
5-Hydroxytryptamine	2.5 ng/ml
Iproniazid	50 μg/ml
Tryptamine	100 ng/ml

Expt. 7.1 Agonists and the rat fundus strip preparation

The preparation is based on the method of Vane (1957). Kill a rat by a blow on the neck and exsanguinate the animal. Open the abdomen and locate the stomach. The fundal part is the upper part of the stomach and easily identifiable by its grey colour. Cut the rest of the stomach away from the fundal region and transfer the fundus to a petri dish containing Ringer solution. Open out the fundal end longitudinally by making two cuts either side of the dome shaped preparation. The tissue should now lie flat in the petri dish. Prepare a strip from the tissue by making alternate transverse cuts on opposite sides of the muscle. It is usually possible to obtain two strips about 4 cm long from each animal. Tie threads around each end of the strip and attach one end to a tissue holder. Transfer the mounted preparation to an organ bath and attach the other thread to the transducer. Apply an additional 1 g stretching weight as described for the frog rectus muscle in Expt. 4.1.

Experimental protocol

1 Show dose related responses to acetylcholine.
2 Repeat 1 for histamine. Do not use concentrations $> 50\,\mu g/ml$.
3 Repeat 1 for 5-hydroxytryptamine.
4 Repeat 1 for tryptamine.
5 Repeat 1 for bradykinin.
6 Add 2-bromolysergic acid diethylamide to the organ bath and leave in contact with the tissue for 20–30 minutes and without washing repeat a dose of 5-hydroxytryptamine which produced a large submaximal response.
7 Replace 2-bromolysergic acid diethylamide in the organ bath and without washing repeat a dose of tryptamine which produced a large submaximal response.
8 Repeat 7 using acetylcholine instead of tryptamine.
9 Repeat 7 using bradykinin instead of tryptamine.

This experiment should show the high sensitivity of rat fundus to 5-hydroxytryptamine and virtually complete insensitivity to histamine. Tryptamine is also an agonist at 5-hydroxytryptamine receptors and lysergic acid diethylamide will antagonise both agonists leaving bradykinin and acetylcholine responses unaffected. It may sometimes be observed that acetylcholine responses are potentiated after 2-bromolysergic acid diethylamide. This may be due to anticholinesterase activity that this compound is reputed to possess.

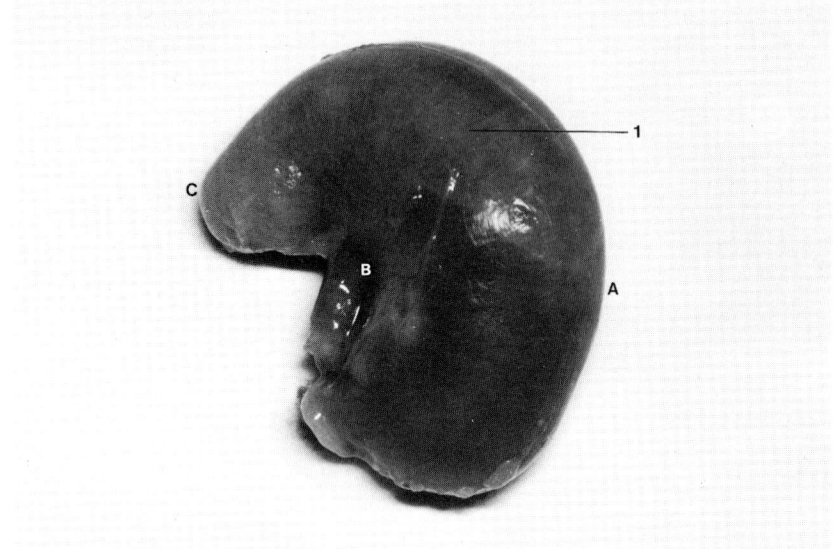

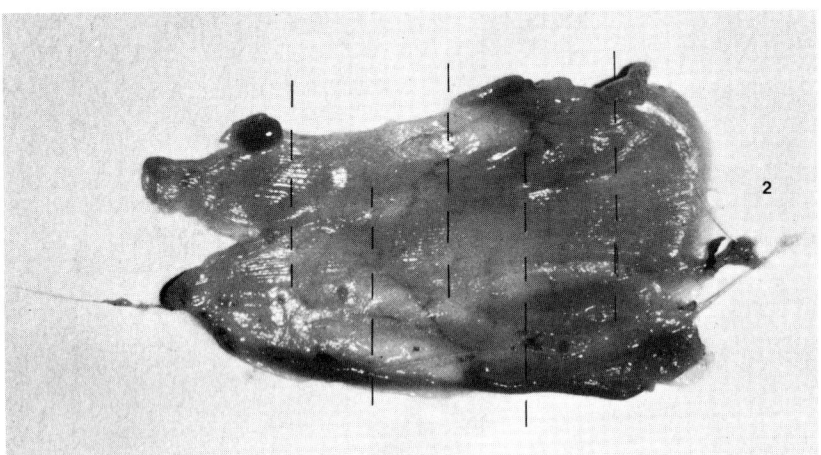

Fig. 34. Dissection of the rat fundus strip.

The fundal region is the upper part of the stomach (1) and is dissected out and opened up flat by making cuts from A to B and B to C. A strip is prepared from the flat muscle preparation (2) by cutting as indicated by the dotted lines.

Consistent responses to both agonists and antagonists take considerable time to develop in the preparation and as long as possible should be left after setting up the tissue and after adding antagonists.

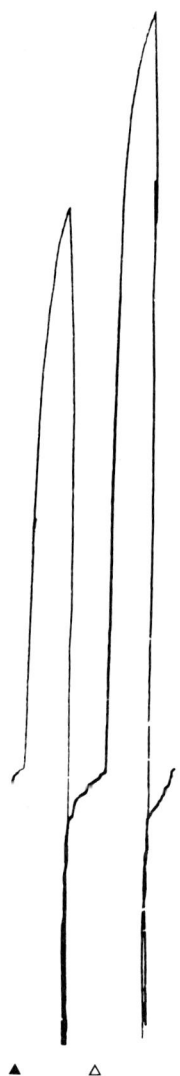

Fig. 35. Responses of the rat fundus strip to 5-hydroxytryptamine (▲ 20 ng/ml, △ 50 ng/ml).

Expt. 7.2 Effect of a monoamine oxidase inhibitor on responses of the rat fundus strip to 5-hydroxytryptamine and tryptamine

Set up the rat fundus as described in Expt. 7.1.

Experimental protocol

1 Show dose related responses to 5-hydroxytryptamine and tryptamine.

2 Add iproniazid to the Ringer reservoir and leave in contact with the tissue for 15 minutes. Repeat 1.

This experiment should show the potentiation of responses to tryptamine produced by monoamine oxidase inhibitors and the lack of effect upon 5-hydroxytryptamine responses.

Miscellaneous
Smooth Muscle Preparations

Introduction

A few smooth muscle preparations which are of use and interest to the pharmacologist do not fall into any of the categories previously described. An introduction to each tissue is given below:

1 Rat anococcygeus muscle.

This preparation, originally described by Gillespie in 1972, has emerged in the last decade as an unusual tissue for pharmacological research and can be successfully studied by undergraduate students. The anococcygeus is a thin strip of smooth muscle which arises from sacral vertebrae and passes over the terminal colon. It is much larger in the male rat than in the female and this has led to speculation that its physiological function is to close off the colon during ejaculation in the male. The muscle receives a dense adrenergic innervation but apparently no cholinergic innervation and stimulation of sympathetic nerves causes contraction of the muscle. However, the anococcygeus is particularly interesting in that it appears to receive a second, non-adrenergic, non-cholinergic inhibitory innervation of which the transmitter is, as yet, unknown. The nerve mediated responses are generated by modified field stimulation. It is usual to locate a ring electrode (identical to that used for the chick biventer cervicis muscle) over the muscle. Neurally evoked contractions can be obtained using this arrangement.

The anococcygeus muscle contracts to noradrenaline, acetylcholine and 5-hydroxytryptamine, isoprenaline at high concentrations but not to histamine. Noradrenaline and acetylcholine effects are blocked by phentolamine and atropine respectively.

2 Guinea-pig tracheal chain.

The trachea comprises a series of incomplete rings of cartilage. The ring is completed by layers of smooth muscle. This muscle behaves like bronchiolar muscle and is therefore useful for demonstrating the β_2-adrenoceptors which predominate in the respiratory system. Its main disadvantage is that it is tedious to prepare the tissue and the responses, as with most respiratory tissues, are slow in onset and offset. β_2-adrenoceptors mediate broncholdilation by stimulating adenyl cylase and releasing cyclic AMP.

3 Guinea-pig taenia caeci.

There are several isolated tissue preparations from the lower part of the intestine which have undergone pharmacological investigation. The terminal colon, of the rat, guinea-pig and mouse are all suitable for practical use by students, but a preparation which has aroused greater interest is the taenia of the guinea-pig caecum. In parts of the large intestine of many species the longitudinally arranged muscle is grouped into bands, called taeniae. The muscle preparation has been commonly called taenia coli, but this is really inappropriate since the longitudinal muscle of the guinea-pig colon is not arranged in taeniae. Like other intestinal muscle both excitatory parasympathetic nerves and inhibitory sympathetic fibres serve the tissue. The taeniae are also innervated by intramural inhibitory nerves with their cell bodies in Auerbach's plexus. These nerves can be excited by electrical stimulation of the taenia or by the application of ganglion-stimulating drugs. The intramural inhibitory nerves have different properties from sympathetic nerves, and it has been suggested that ATP or a related nucleotide is the transmitter substance released from the non-adrenergic nerves.

Stimulation of sympathetic nerves can be effected by perivascular stimulation as for jejunal preparations (see Expt. 2.4). The inhibitory responses to perivascular stimulation are abolished by adrenergic neurone blockers. In contrast, responses to field stimulation are unaffected by guanethidine but can be shown to be neuronally mediated.

The preparation requires a long equilibration period and even after this, tone may vary from preparation to preparation. When the tone is low, spontaneous beats of relatively large amplitude may be observed. Noradrenaline will inhibit the beats but often does not produce appreciable relaxation. More commonly the tone is high and the spontaneous beats are more irregular and of smaller amplitude. This type of preparation is most desirable for Expt. 8.3 In some preparations relaxations induced by stimulation are followed by an after contraction which may persist for up to 1 minute.

Experimental parameters

Organ bath	Anococcygeus	20 ml
	Tracheal chain	10 ml
	Taenia caeci	50 ml

Ringer solution	Anococcygeus/trachea	Krebs
	Taenia caeci	McEwens
Aeration		95% O_2/5% CO_2
Bath temperature	Anococcygeus/trachea	37°C
	Taenia caeci	35°C
Recording	Anococcygeus/trachea	Isometric
	Taenia caeci	Isotonic
Resting tension	Anococcygeus/trachea	0.5 g
	Taenia caeci	1 g
Equilibration period	Anococcygeus	30 minutes
	Tracheal chain	45 minutes
	Taenia caeci	45–60 minutes
Dose cycle	Anococcygeus	3–5 minutes
	Tracheal chain	20 minutes
	Taenia caeci	5 minutes
Contact time	Anococcygeus	$1\frac{1}{2}$–2 minutes
	Tracheal chain	2 minutes
Stimulus parameters	Expt. 8.1	Pulse width 0.5 ms
		Voltage 30 V
		Frequency 1–50 Hz
		Stimulus duration 1–2 minutes
	Expt. 8.3 (perivascular stimulation)	Pulse width 2 ms
		Voltage 20 V
		Frequency 1–40 Hz
		Stimulus duration 10 s
	Expt. 8.3 (field stimulation)	Pulse width 0.5 ms
		Voltage 40 V (> 50 mA)
		Frequency 1–40 Hz
		Stimulus duration 10 s

Drugs (final bath concentration: starting dose)

	Annococcygeus	Tracheal chain	Taenia caeci
Cocaine	500 ng/ml		
Guanethidine	100 μg/ml		1 μg/ml
Isoprenaline		5 ng/ml	
Noradrenaline	50 ng/ml		5 ng/ml
Practolol		150 ng/ml	

	Annococcygeus	Tracheal chain	Taenia caeci
Propranolol		100 ng/ml	
Salbutamol		30 ng/ml	
Tetrodotoxin	500 ng/ml		1 μg/ml

Expt. 8.1 Drugs and the field-stimulated anococcygeus muscle of the rat

The preparation is based on the method of Gillespie (1972). Kill a rat by a blow on the neck and exsanguinate the animal. Open the abdomen and move the lower part of the intestine to one side. Remove the bladder and urethra. Raise the pelvis with forceps and split the pelvis along the mid-line using a pair of scissors. Force the bone apart to reveal the terminal colon. Cut the colon 1–2 cm from the anal margin. Lift the colon and carefully clear the surrounding connective tissue towards the anus until the two anococcygeus muscles (about 1–2 cm in length) can be identified. They arise from the vertebrae and can be followed at an acute angle to their point of meeting over

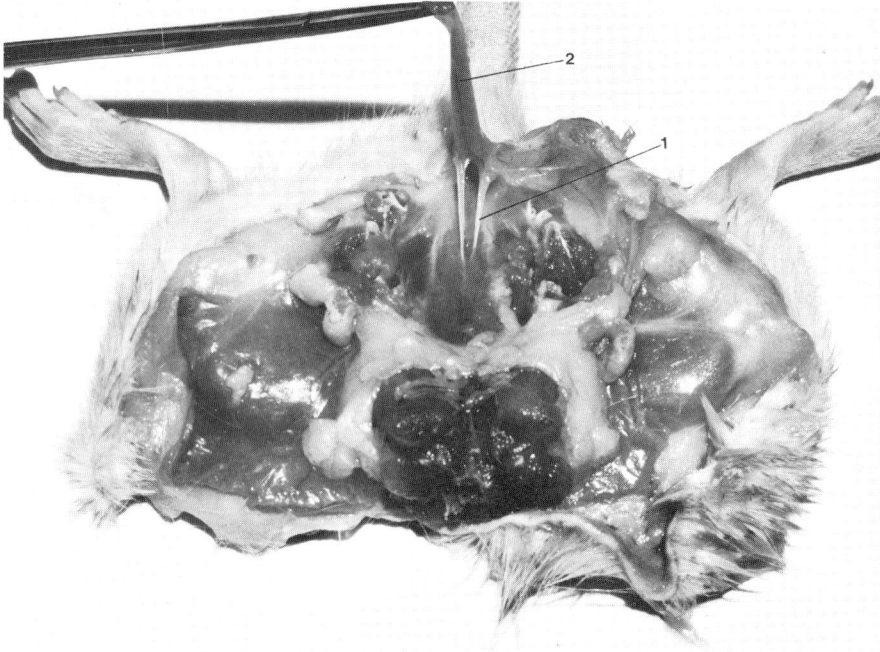

Fig. 36. Dissection of the rat anococcygeus muscles.
Ties are placed around the muscles (1) where they emerge from the spinal cord and dissected out to their point of attachment to the terminal colon (2).

the terminal colon. It is sometimes easy to confuse the anococcygeus muscles and the connective tissue surrounding the colon. A bright dissecting light aids the identification of the muscles which are an opaque white colour. Ensure that the muscles are kept moist with Ringer. Clear one muscle of connective tissue and tie a thread around the tendonous region close to the spine. Cut the muscle free from the spine and using the thread to apply minimal tension follow the muscle back to the ventral side of the colon. Tie a second thread as close to the point of attachment to the colon as possible and remove the muscle from the animal. The second muscle can be similarly prepared and two preparations can be obtained from each rat. Tie a loop at one end of the muscle and attach this to a tissue holder. Transfer the preparation to an organ bath. Pass the other thread through a ring electrode and secure the electrode centrally around the muscle. Attach the upper thread to the transducer.

Experimental protocol

1 Show dose related responses to noradrenaline.
2 Show frequency-related responses to field stimulation.
3 Add cocaine to the bath and leave in contact for 5 minutes. Without washing add a dose of noradrenaline that produced a response about 50% of maximal in 1.
4 Repeat 3 for a 50% of maximal field-stimulated response instead of noradrenaline.
5 Show field-stimulated responses to 10 Hz stimulation using a 3 minute dose cycle. Add guanethidine to the bath and continue stimulating at 3 minute intervals without washing until reproducible inhibitory responses are obtained.
6 Add tetrodotoxin and continue stimulating until inhibitory responses are abolished.

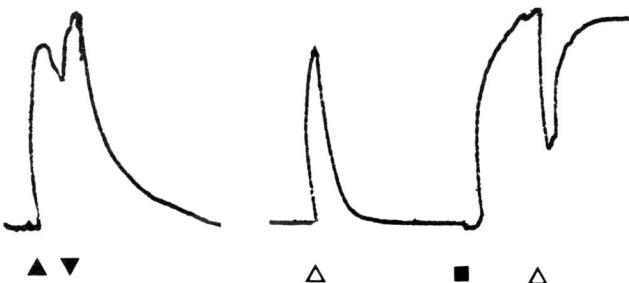

Fig. 37. Responses of the rat anococcygeus muscle to noradrenaline (▲ 150 ng/ml ▼ wash), field stimulation (△ 10 Hz, 1 min), and to guanethidine (■ 60 μg/ml).

This experiment should show the parallel between field-stimulated responses and exogenous noradrenaline administration. Both are potentiated by block of neuronal reuptake with cocaine. Stimulated responses are abolished by an adrenergic neurone blocker such as guanethidine, and with time the tone of the muscle increases and inhibitory responses to field stimulation are observed. If time permits the putative neurotransmitter involved in this response can be studied by showing the effects of various known antagonists. The above experiment shows that this inhibitory effect is neuronally mediated as tetrodotoxin eventually abolishes the response.

Expt. 8.2 The nature of adrenoceptors in the guinea-pig tracheal chain preparation

The preparation is based on the method of Castillo and De Beer (1947). Kill a guinea-pig by dislocating the neck. If the animal is exsanguinated, take care to cut the throat as high up as possible to avoid damage to the trachea. Open the neck and upper thorax and clear the muscles surrounding the trachea. Dissect out a length of at least 6 cm trachea and place the tissue in cold oxygenated Krebs Ringer in a petri dish. Cut at least 6 rings of muscle from the trachea by making transverse cuts. Each ring should contain not more than two bands of cartilage. The rings are D-shaped and it is the straight part of the D which consists of smooth muscle. Tie the rings together with fine thread attached to the cartilage so that the smooth muscle is in the longitudinal plane and each alternate ring has muscle on opposite sides. Make the ties between rings as close to the smooth muscle as possible. Sometimes the D-shape is not very clear but the cartilage can usually be identified as it is an opaque white colour. Cut through the cartilage of each ring between the ties and attach one end of the chain to a tissue holder. Transfer the mounted tissue to an organ bath and attach the upper thread to the transducer. Allow drugs to act for 2 minutes and wash out the bath. A period of 20 minutes is usually required between doses and during this time the tissue should not be kept under tension.

Experimental protocol

1   Add salbutamol.
2   Add isoprenaline.
3   Add practolol and leave in contact with the tissue for 15 minutes. Repeat 1 and 2 and replace practolol in the organ bath after washing the tissue.

4 Wash out practolol and re-establish responses to 1 and 2.

5 Repeat 3 using propranolol instead of practolol.

The relaxant effects of salbutamol and isoprenaline should be observed in this preparation. Both responses are mediated predominantly through β_2-adrenoceptors and blocked by propranolol. β_1-adrenoceptors will probably not be present and practolol (a selective β_1-antagonist) is unlikely to affect reponses to the mixed β_1/β_2-agonist isoprenaline.

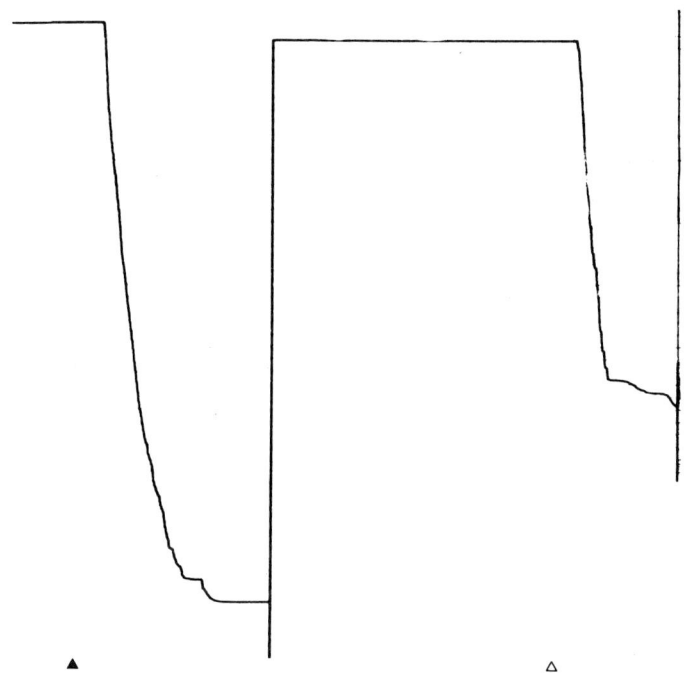

Fig. 38. Responses of the guinea-pig tracheal chain to isoprenaline (▲ 20 ng/ml, △ 10 ng/ml).

Expt. 8.3 Inhibitory responses of the taenia caeci of the guinea-pig to perivascular and field stimulation

The preparation is based on the method of Burnstock et al. (1965). Kill a guinea-pig by dislocating the neck and exsanguinate the animal. Locate the caecum and identify the three bands of taeniae. They run in the longitudinal plane and are easily identified as greyish strips of muscle. It is easiest to use the taenia which lies on the underneath surface of the caecum. The caecum should be turned over to expose the ileo-caecal angle and the lymph node that lies in the angle. Identify the large blood vessel lying between the terminal ileum and the caecum and follow this vessel over the lymph node to its branches over the caecal wall and to the taenia. Using a needle pass a thread

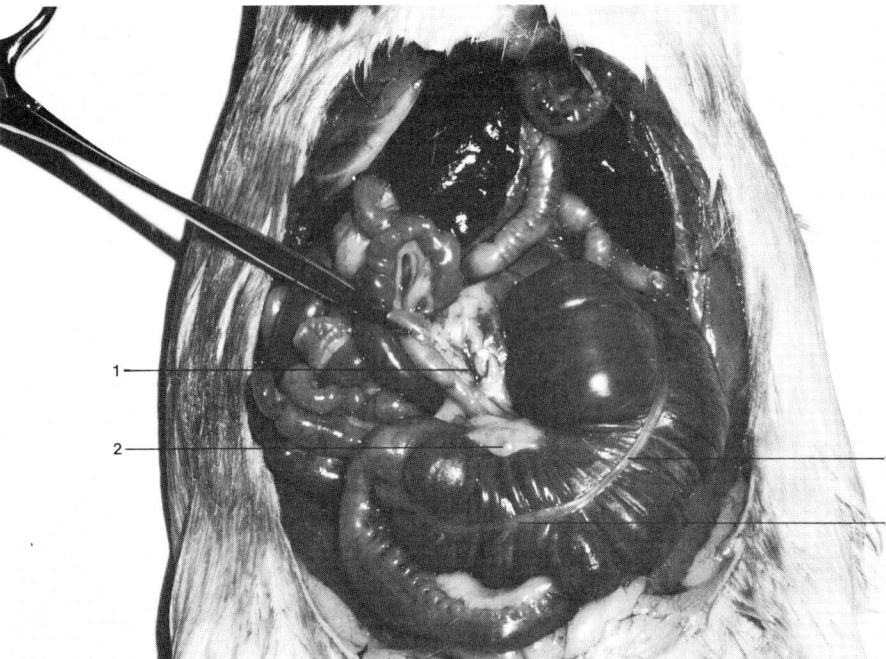

Fig. 39. Dissection of the guinea-pig taenia caeci.

A tie is placed around the perivascular supply (1) and dissected out towards the lymph node (2) and the taenia. Ties are made at the points indicated (3).

of cotton underneath the vascular supply to the tissue about 3–4 cm from the ileo-caecal angle. Tie the thread around the vessel and dissect out the vascular supply towards the tissue. Keep the preparation moist at all times. Using a needle pass a thread of cotton underneath the taenia about 2 cm from the central point of attachment of the blood vessel. Tie the thread firmly around the muscle, leaving sufficient cotton for attachment, at a later stage, to the transducer. Tie a second thread about 4 cm from the first ensuring that the entry of the vascular supply to the muscle lies between the two threads. Leave sufficient cotton for attachment to the tissue holder. Dissect out the taenia using one thread to apply tension to the muscle to aid its removal. Take care not to damage the muscle. It is often best to remove a small amount of the surrounding circular muscle tissue. Transfer the preparation to a petri dish containing McEwen's Ringer. Trim excessive connective tissue from the blood vessel but do not be over zealous with this procedure. Tie one end of the muscle to the tissue holder and transfer the preparation to an organ bath set up for field stimulation. Locate the blood vessel in a jaw electrode or pull the vessel through a Saxby electrode and secure the electrode alongside the tissue in a manner similar to that described for the Finkleman preparation (Expt. 2.4). Attach the upper thread from the muscle to the transducer. Ensure that the electrode does not interfere with muscle movement or the field stimulation electrodes.

Experimental protocol

1   Show frequency related inhibitory responses to perivascular stimulation (1–40 Hz). Do not wash the tissue between stimulation.
2   Repeat 1 for field stimulation.
3   Show dose-related inhibition of intestinal movements by carrying out a dose-response curve to noradrenaline.

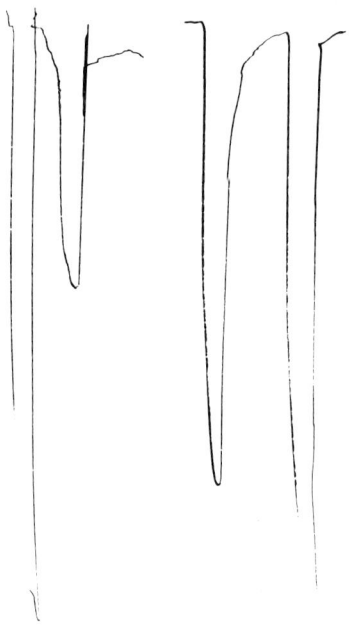

Fig. 40. Responses of the guinea-pig taenia caeci to perivascular stimulation (▲ 50 Hz; △ 30 Hz) and noradrenaline (■ 5 ng/ml; □ 20 ng/ml).

4 Add guanethidine to the Ringer solution and leave the tissue to equilbriate for 5 minutes.

5 Repeat 1.

6 Repeat 2.

7 Repeat 3.

8 Add tetrodotoxin to the Ringer solution and leave the tissue to equilibrate for 5 minutes.

9 Repeat 2.

The experiment should show relaxations induced by noradrenaline and comparable inhibitory reponses produced by perivascular and field stimulation. The adrenergic neurone blocker should abolish responses to perivascular stimulation and may potentiate response to exogenous noradrenaline due to block of neuronal re-uptake. In contrast field stimulated responses should be unaffected and can be abolished by tetrodotoxin.

If contractile reponses are observed at low frequencies of stimulation the contractile effects of acetylcholine and the inhibitory effects of atropine can be investigated.

Miscellaneous Experiments

The following section includes a number of experiments which cannot easily be classified into the previous sections. Each experiment is considered separately and is preceded by an introduction.

Expt. 9.1 Local anaesthetics and the foot-withdrawal reflex of the frog

Introduction

The activity of local anaesthetic drugs in practical pharmacology can be demonstrated in several ways. In man, the blocking of needle prick sensations on the forearm can be shown by intradermal injections of local anaesthetics. A similar method can be employed in guinea-pigs using the intradermal injections on the shaved back of the animal and a squeak or twitch in response to needle pricks is interpreted as an indication of pain sensation. It is also possible to demonstrate local anaesthetic activity *in vitro* using the sciatic nerve block technique in the frog. Decapitated, pithed and eviscerated frogs are hung from a cork board and the reflex withdrawal of the feet when dipped into acid is monitored. The screening method involves block of axonal conduction and if local anaesthetics are placed in the eviscerated pouch, block of conduction in the sciatic nerves results and the reflex is abolished. The method can therefore be used to assess the time of onset of local anaesthetics.

All local anaesthetics belong to the class of membrane stabilising drugs. Two are investigated in this experiment, procaine and amethocaine. Amethocaine is more potent than procaine and has a faster onset of action.

Method

Kill a frog by stunning and decapitate the animal. Pith only the upper part of the spinal cord, if desired. The procedure is often not necessary. Remove the exposed viscera from the abdominal pouch with fine forceps taking care not to damage the nerves at the base of the spinal cord. Pin the frog by its front

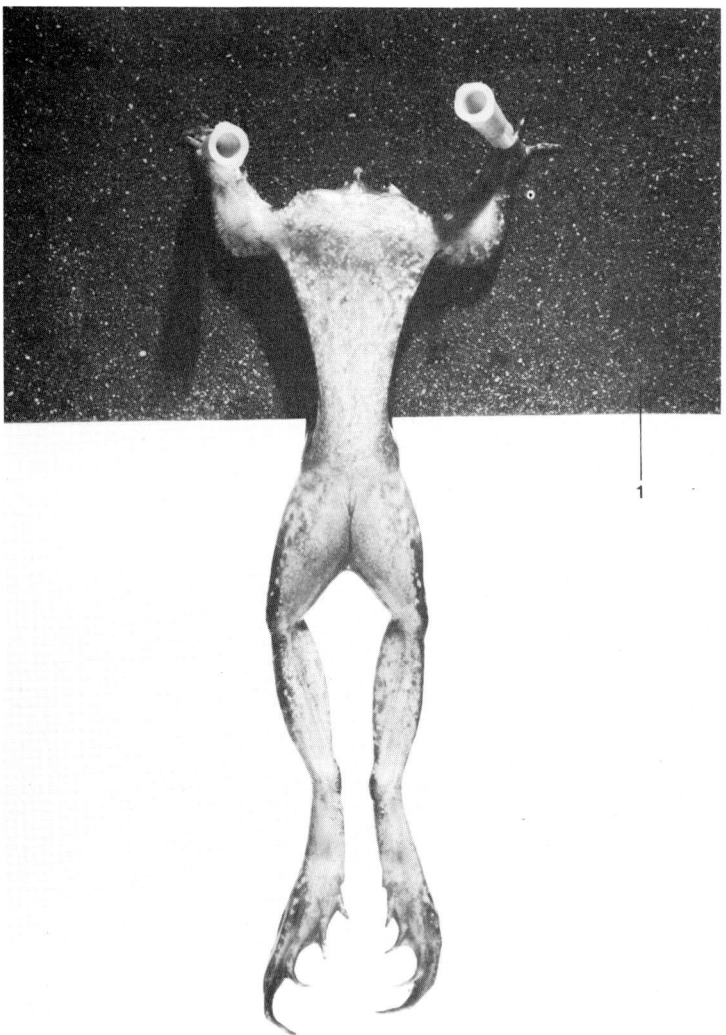

Fig. 41. Mounting of eviscerated frog for foot-withdrawal reflex.

An eviscerated frog is pinned to a cork board (1) and the legs allowed to hang free below the board for immersion in dilute HCl in order to test the foot-withdrawal reflex.

limbs to a vertically mounted cork board so that the hind legs are suspended freely below it. It is important that the experiment is begun immediately.

Experimental protocol

1 Dip both hind ligs into a beaker containing 0.05 M HCl and note the time taken for the frog to withdraw the foot. If no response is observed after 10 seconds try 0.1 M HCl. If this is ineffective exclude the frog from the experiment.

2 Immediately following a response (i.e. foot withdrawal) wash the legs by immersing in a beaker of 0.6% saline and rinsing with a saline wash bottle.

3 Introduce 1 ml of the local anaesthetic to be tested into the abdominal pouch and start the stopclock.

4 Test at 1 minute intervals the foot withdrawal reflex using the lowest concentration of HCl that illicits a response. If a response is not observed increase the HCl concentration (0.05 M to 0.1 M to 0.2 M). The end point (i.e. a full local anaesthetic effect) is taken as failure to remove the feet from 0.2 M HCl after 10 seconds contact.

5 Repeat 3 and 4 for at least three concentrations of amethocaine and procaine using a new frog for each determination.

It is recommended that concentrations of amethocaine (500 μg–2.5 mg) and procaine (1 mg–5 mg) are used. The onset of block needs to be observed between 2 and 20 minutes since the reflex often only last for 30 minutes.

Data from each student participating in the practical should be collated and means and standard errors for onset of anaesthesia calculated. Statistical analysis should then be performed on this data. Note however that the response is quite variable and markedly dependent on the experimenter's ability to produce consistent preparations.

Expt. 9.2 Effect of sodium cromoglycate on compound 48/80 induced release of histamine from isolated peritoneal mast cells of the rat

Introduction

Release of histamine from mast cells can be effected in several ways. Stores of histamine in peripheral tissues can be depleted by the potent histamine releaser polymer, compound 48/80. The prophylactic anti-asthmatic drug, sodium cromoglycate owes part of its therapeutic effect to its ability to act as a mast cell stabiliser. It blocks degranulation of mast cells and the release of histamine induced by compound 48/80.

The time of addition of sodium cromoglycate is critical. Maximum inhibition is usually obtained when compound 48/80 and sodium cromoglycate are added together and inhibition is most marked using low doses of compound 48/80. Possibly histamine release by low concentrations occurs by a selective release of amine containing granules through a process of exocytosis, as does the reagin-induced histamine release from sensitised mast cells.

Method

Set up a guinea-pig ileum preparation as described in Expt. 2.1.

Kill five rats by a blow on the neck and exsanguinate the animals. Immediately inject 4 mls of heparinised Tyrodes Ringer (5 units/ml) intraperitoneally and massage the abdomen for 1 minute. Open the abdomen and remove the Tyrodes with a plastic syringe. Ensure the solutions are clear of blood and pool the solution in a plastic tube. Keep the mast cell suspension on ice. If the solution is not clear centrifuge at 300 g for 5 minutes, discard the supernatant and resuspend the pellet in Tyrodes (20 ml).

Set up plastic centrifuge tubes (in duplicate) for incubation in accordance with the following table but do not add the mast cell suspension until you are ready to begin your timed incubations.

Tube No.	Tyrode only	48/80 in Tyrode μg/ml					Sodium cromoglycate in Tyrode μg/ml		Mast cell suspension
		0.2	0.4	1.0	2.0	4.0	20	40	
1	1 ml	–	–	–	–	–	–	–	1 ml
2	–	1 ml	–	–	–	–	–	–	1 ml
3	–	–	–	1 ml	–	–	–	–	1 ml
4	–	–	–	–	1 ml	–	–	–	1 ml
5	–	–	0.5 ml	–	–	–	–	0.5 ml	1 ml
6	–	–	–	–	0.5 ml	–	–	0.5 ml	1 ml
7	–	–	–	–	–	0.5 ml	–	0.5 ml	1 ml
8	–	–	–	–	–	–	1 ml	–	1 ml
9	1 ml	–	–	–	–	–	–	–	1 ml

Experimental protocol

1 Incubate tubes 1–8 at 37°C for 15 minutes. Centrifuge at 200 g (1300 r.p.m. using a bench centrifuge) for 10 minutes. Decant the resulting supernatant for assay leaving the cells as a pellet in the tube.

2 Boil tube 9 for 15 minutes. Place a marble over the tube to prevent evaporation. Centrifuge and treat as 1.

3 Assay each supernatant against histamine using a bracket assay on the guinea-pig ileum (see p. 55).

4 Show that both the responses to histamine and to supernatants are antagonised by diphenhydramine (100 ng/ml).

The experiment should provide the following information:

1 spontaneous release of histamine from mast cells (Tube 1);

2 total histamine content of mast cells (released by boiling—Tube 9);

3 concentration dependent release of histamine by compound 48/80 (Tubes 2–4);

4 inhibition of compound 48/80 induced histamine release by sodium cromoglycate (Tubes 5–7);

5 effect of sodium cromoglycate on spontaneous release of histamine (Tube 8).

The percentage net release of histamine by compound 48/80 should be calculated. At the highest dose it is likely to be some 80% of the total histamine content, and only about 20% in the presence of sodium cromoglycate. Sodium cromoglycate does not inhibit or potentiate the spontaneous release of histamine. Antagonism of the supernatant responses by an H_1-antagonist should confirm that histamine is being measured.

Expt. 9.3 Effect of tubocurarine and morphine on histamine release from rat skin, muscle and lung mast cells

Introduction

Early studies of histamine release were performed *in vivo* but it was realised that *in vitro* experiments were of value when it was demonstrated that tubocurarine released histamine from the isolated rat diaphragm. Some drugs, e.g. morphine, tubocurarine and guanethidine release histamine and this side effect can be undesirable in the therapeutic use of these agents. These drugs are able to release histamine from a number of tissues and this effect is demonstrated in this experiment.

Method

Set up an isolated guinea-pig ileum preparation as described in Expt. 2.1.

Kill two rats by a blow on the neck and exsanguinate the animals. Shave the abdomen and remove the abdominal skin. Trim off any subcutaneous fat. Open the thoracic cavity and remove the lungs and the diaphragm. Chop the tissues into approximately 2 mm square pieces with fine scissors and wash with warm incubating medium (NaCl 9.1 g/l, KCl 2.0 g/l, CaCl$_2$ 0.1 g/l, 100 ml phosphate buffer). Divide the chopped tissue into three equal portions by weight.

Experimental protocol

1 Place the three tissue portions into plastic tubes containing 5 ml of incubating medium.
2 Incubate for 5 minutes at 37°C and remove solution for assay as described in Expt. 9.2.3.
3 Replace the solution with
a) 5 ml of incubating medium
b) 5 ml of incubating medium + morphine (100 μg/ml)
c) 5 ml of incubating medium + tubocurarine (1 mg/ml) and incubate for 1 h at 37°C.
4 Remove solutions and assay as for 2.
5 Boil tissue residue with 0.1 M HCl (3 ml) for 10 minutes. Neutralise with 0.1 M NaOH and centrifuge as for Expt. 9.2.
6 Assay as before.

Histamine release should be expressed in relation to tissue weight and the remaining tissue histamine content can be determined from the assay of 5.

Expt. 9.4 The use of parallel comparative bioassay

Introduction

The use of parallel comparative bioassay (or parallel assay for short) is still an important part of pharmacological research. The principle can be employed in two ways:
1 to be certain that the identity of a substance in an extract matches that of a known standard. The activity of the standard against the activity of the extract is compared on two or more tissues. If the unknown and standard are identical then the potency ratio on each tissue should vary in parallel;
2 to indicate if different agonists (within a series of compounds) mediate

their effects through different receptors in different isolated tissues. If a series of agonists act upon the same receptor in two tissue preparations then the relative potency ratios between agonists should be identical.

Principle 2 is investigated in the following experiment. Opioid agonists mediate their effects via multiple opioid receptor sites and the distribution of these receptor sites varies from one opioid-sensitive tissue preparation to another. For example, the mouse vas deferens contains predominantly δ-opioid receptors whilst the guinea-pig ileum has a predominantly μ-opioid receptor population. μ-receptor agonists are more potent at inhibiting the field-stimulated guinea-pig ileum preparation than the field-stimulated mouse vas deferens. In contrast δ-receptor agonists are more potent in the vas than in the ileum. This disparity between potency ratios was originally used to suggest the existence of multiple opioid receptor sites.

Method

Set up a field-stimulated guinea-pig ileum preparation and a field stimulated mouse vas deferens preparation as described in Expt. 2.5 and Expt. 5.2. respectively.

Experimental protocol

For both preparations show:
1 A full dose-response curve to morphine.
2 A full dose-response curve to leu-enkephalin.

Calculate the IC_{50} value for morphine and leu-enkephalin (i.e. the concentration of agonist producing 50% inhibition of the twitch responses) using linear regression of points between 20 and 80% of maximum.

A comparison of the potency ratios for each opioid on the two preparations should indicate that their effects are mediated via different receptor systems.

Bibliography

Introduction

References

Bennett A. and Stockley H. L. (1974) Effect of electrode positions on contractions of guinea-pig isolated ileum to electrical stimulation. *Br. J. Pharmac.* **50,** 453P.

Burn J. H. & Rand M. J. (1960) The relation of circulating noradrenaline to the effect of sympathetic stimulation. *J. Physiol. (Lond.)* **150,** 295–305.

Edinburgh University Pharmacology Staff (1968) *Pharmacological Experiments on Isolated Preparations.* Churchill Livingstone.

Harper B. & Hughes I. E. (1978) The effect of stimulus intensity on α-adrenoceptor-mediated feedback control of noradrenaline release. *Br. J. Pharmac.* **63,** 689–691.

Further reading

Paton W. D. M. (1954) The response of the guinea-pig ileum to electrical stimulation by coaxial electrodes. *J. Physiol. (Lond.)* **127,** 40–41P.

Sperelakis N. (1962) Contraction of depolarised muscle by electric fields. *Am. J. Physiol.* **202,** 731–742.

Van Rossom J. M. (1963) Cumulative dose-response curves. II. Technique for the making of dose-response curves in isolated organs and the evaluation of drug parameters. *Arch int. Pharmacodyn.* **143,** 299–330.

Isolated uterus

Reference

De Jalon, Bayo & De Jalon (1945) *Farmacoter.* act **3,** 313.

Further reading

Vane J. R. & Williams K. I. (1973) The contribution of prostaglandin production to contractions of the isolated uterus of the rat. *Br. J. Pharmac.* **48,** 629–639.

Isolated small intestine (Qualitative experiments)

References

Gaddum J.H. & Picarelli Z.P. (1957) Two kinds of tryptamine receptor. *Br. J. Pharmac.* **12,** 323-328.

Finkleman B. (1930) On the nature of inhibition in the intestine. *J. Physiol. (Lond.)* **70,** 145-157.

Handa B.K., Lane A.C., Lord J.A.H., Morgan B.A., Rance M.J. & Smith C.F.C. (1981) Analogues of β-LPH$_{61-64}$ possessing selective agonist activity at μ-opiate receptors. *Eur. J. Pharmac.* **70,** 531-540.

Holman M.E. & Hughes J.R. (1965) Inhibition of intestinal smooth muscle. *Aust. J. exp. Biol. med. Sci.* **43,** 277-290.

Magnus (1904) *Pflügers Arch ges Physiol.* **102,** 123.

Paton W.D.M. & Zar M. Aboo (1968) The origin of acetylcholine released from guinea-pig intestine and longitudinal muscle strips. *J. Physiol.* **194,** 13-33.

Rang H.P. (1964) Stimulant actions of volatile anaesthetics on smooth muscle. *Br. J. Pharmac.* **22,** 356-365.

Isolated small intenstine (Quantitative experiments)

Reference

Lockett M.S. & Bartlett A.L. (1956) A method for the determination of pA$_2$ at two minutes. *J. Pharm. Pharmac.* **8,** 18-26.

Further reading

Arunlakshana O. & Schild H.O. (1959) Some quantitative uses of drug antagonists. *Br. J. Pharmac.* **14,** 48-58.

Gaddum J.H. (1937) The quantitative effects of antagonistic drugs. *J. Physiol.* **89,** 7P.

Furchgott R.F. (1966) The use of β-haloalkylamines in the differentiation of receptors and in the determination of dissocation constants of receptor agonist complexes. *Adv. Drug Res.* **3,** 21-56.

Nickerson M. (1956) Receptor occupancy and tissue response. *Nature* **178,** 697-698.

Schild H.O. (1947) pA, a new scale for the measurement of drug antagonism. *Br. J. Pharmac.* **2,** 189-206.

Stephenson R.P. (1956) A modification of receptor theory. *Br. J. Pharmac.* **11,** 379-393.

Isolated skeletal muscle

References

Bulbring E. (1946) Observations on the isolated phrenic nerve diaphragm preparation of the rat. *Br. J. Pharmac.* **1,** 38-61.

Ginsborg B.L. & Warriner J. (1960) The isolated chick biventer cervicis nerve muscle preparation. *Br. J. Pharmac.* **15,** 410-416.

Further reading

Bowman W.C. & Nott M.W. (1969) Actions of sympathomimetic amines and their antagonists on skeletal muscle. *Pharmac. Rev.* **21**, 27–72.

Miyamoto M.D. (1978) The actions of cholinergic drugs on motor nerve terminals. *Pharmac. Rev.* **29**, 221–247.

Zaimis E. (ed.) (1976) Neuromuscular junction. *Handb. Exp. Pharmac.* **42**, Springer-Verlag, Berlin.

Isolated vas deferens

References

Hart S.L., Kitchen I. & Waddell P.R. (1979) Different effects of current strength on inhibitory responses of the mouse vas deferens to methionine- and leucine-enkephalin. *Br. J. Pharmac.* **66**, 361–363.

Henderson G., Hughes J. & Kosterlitz H.W. (1972) A new example of a morphine sensitive neuro-effector junction: adrenergic transmission in the mouse vas deferens. *Br. J. Pharmac.* **46** 764–766.

Hukovic S. (1961) Responses of the isolated nerve-ductus deferens preparation of the guinea-pig. *Br. J. Pharmac.* **16**, 188–194.

Further reading

Ambache N., Dunk L.P., Verney J. & Zar M. Aboo (1972) Inhibition of postganglionic motor transmission in vas deferens by indirectly acting sympathomimetic drugs. **227**, 433–456.

Ambache N. & Zar M. Aboo (1971) Evidence against adrenergic transmission in the guinea-pig vas deferens. *J. Physiol. (Lond.)* **216**, 359–389.

Brown C.M., McGrath J.C. & Summers R.J. (1979) The effects of α-adrenoceptor agonists and antagonists on responses of transmurally stimulated prostatic and epididymal portions of the isolated vas deferens of the rat. *Br. J. Pharmac.* **66**, 553–564.

Kosterlitz H.W. & Watt A.J. (1968) Kinetic parameters of narcotic agonists and antagonists, with particular reference to N-allylnoroxymorphone (naloxone). *Br. J. Pharmac.* **33**, 266–276.

McKnight A.T., Corbett A.D., Paterson S.J. & Kosterlitz H.W. (1983) Increase in potencies of opioid peptides after peptidase inhibition. *Eur. J. Pharmac.* **86**, 393–402.

Starke K. (1977) Regulation of noradrenaline release by pre-synaptic receptor systems. *Rev. Physiol. Biochem. Pharmac.* **77**, 1–124.

Waterfield A.A., Lord J.A.H., Hughes J. & Kosterlitz H.W. (1978) Differences in the inhibitory effects of normorphine and opioid peptides on the responses of the vasa deferentia of two strains of mice. *Eur. J. Pharmac.* **47**, 249–250.

Cardiac and vascular preparations

References

Furchgott R.F. & Bhadrakom S. (1953) Reactions of strips of rabbit aorta to epinephrine, isopropylarterenol, sodium nitrite and other drugs. *J. Pharmac. exp. Ther.* **108**, 129–143.

Langendorff (1895) *Pflugers Arch ges Physiol.* **190**, 280.

McGregor D.D. (1965) The effect of sympathetic nerve stimulation on the vasconstrictor responses in perfused mesenteric blood vessels of the rat. *J. Physiol. (Lond.)* **177**, 21–30.

Further reading

Burn J.H. & Rand M.J. (1965) Acetylcholine in adrenergic transmission. *Ann. Rev. Pharmac.* **5**, 163–182.

Hirschowitz B.I. (1979) H-2 histamine receptors. *Ann Rev. Pharmac. Toxicol.* **19**, 203–244.

McEwen L.M. (1956) The effect on the isolated rabbit heart of vagal stimulation and its modification by cocaine, hexamethonium and ouabain. *J. Physiol.* **131**, 678–689.

Isolated stomach

Reference

Vane J.R. (1957) A sensitive method for the assay of 5-hydroxytryptamine. *Br. J. Pharmac.* **12**, 344–349.

Further reading

Vane J.R. (1959) The relative activities of some tryptamine analogues on the isolated rat stomach strip preparation. *Br. J. Pharmac.* **14**, 87–98.

Miscellaneous smooth muscle preparations

References

Burnstock G., Campbell G. & Rand M.J. (1966) The inhibitory innervation of the taenia of the guinea-pig caecum. *J. Physiol.* **182**, 504–526.

Castillo J.C. & De Beer E.J. (1947) The tracheal chain. I. A preparation for the study of antispasmodics with particular reference to bronchodilator drugs. *J. Pharmac. exp. Ther.* **90**, 104–109.

Gillespie J.S. (1972) The rat anococcygeus and its response to nerve stimulation and to some drugs. *Br. J. Pharmac.* **45**, 404–416.

Further reading

Burnstock G. (1972) Purinergic nerves. *Pharmacol. Rev.* **24,** 509-581.
Burnstock G., Campbell G., Satchell D. & Smythe A. (1970) Evidence that adenosine triphosphate or a related nucleotide is the transmitter substance released by non-adrenergic inhibitory nerves in the gut. *Br. J. Pharmac.* **40,** 668-688.

Miscellaneous experiments

Further reading

Bulbring E. & Wajda I. (1945) Biological comparison of local anaesthetics. *J. Pharmac. exp. Ther.* **85,** 78-84.
Lord J.A.H., Waterfield A.A., Hughes J. & Kosterlitz H.W. (1977) Endogenous opioid peptides: multiple agonists and receptors. *Nature* **267,** 495-499.
Mongar J.L. & Schild H.O. (1952) A comparison of the effects of anaphylactic shock and of chemical histamine releasers. *J. Physiol. (Lond.)* **118,** 461-478.
Orr T.S.C., Hall D.E., Gwillam J.M. & Cox J.S.G. (1971) The effect of disodium cromoglycate on the release of histamine and degranulation of rat mast cells induced by compound 48/80. *Life Sci.* **10,** 805-812.

Index